Maternity Reflexology Manual

Susanne Enzer

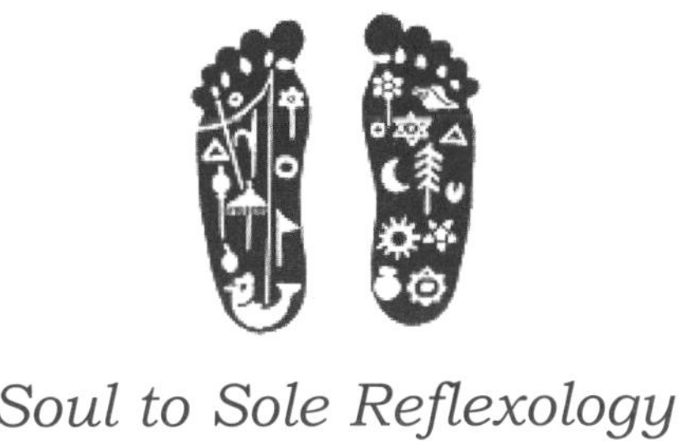

Soul to Sole Reflexology

Maternity Reflexology Manual

Author Susanne Enzer
Production Kate Enzer
Design Susanne Enzer
Photography Adrian Thomas
Illustrations Susanne Enzer

Published in England, 2004 by Soul to Sole Reflexology Ltd.

Printed and bound in England by Hart Press.

ISBN: 0-9548060
1. Reflexology
2. Maternity Care
3. Natural Health Care

For further information regarding his manual contact the author and publisher:
Susanne Enzer, Soul to Sole Reflexology
Email: susanne_enzer@hotmail.com

Note to the reader
Maternity Refelxology Manual is designed as a guide for reflexologists who work with maternity clients. It suggests a complementary health support for maternity clients and is not a substitute for obstetric or medical care.

Acknowledgements

I wish to acknowledge and thank every one who has helped and supported me throughout the creation of this manual:

Firstly, my wonderful sister Erica Greenop who has tirelessly and endlessly supported me when my creative element was flowing and encouraged me when it all seemed "too hard" and never for one moment gave up on me. Her gentle wisdom, her skills with words and above all her love for me has been my mainstay. Thank you.

My beloved daughter, Kate, who has contributed her many skills to turn a workbook into a text book. I am so thrilled with the product - thank you Kate.

Kristine McClure has had a great input in the design co-ordination of the new look Maternity Reflexology, which includes the cover design for this manual and the beautiful Pregnancy Care Reference cards - thank you Kristine.

Lyndall Mollart and Bernadette Leiser, two accomplished, experienced midwives. I thank you not only for your friendship but also for keeping me up-to-date with changes in midwifery.

Throughout the text "What Elsa says" are gentle words of wisdom from the co-author of Maternity Reflexology a Guide for Reflexologists, by Elsa Reid and Susanne Enzer. Reproduced here with Elsa's blessings. Thank you Elsa

Many of the diagrams are taken from my book, Reflexology, a Tool for Midwives and were designed by Jane Charlton. Thank you Jane.

The diagrams and information about the physical development of the Incoming Soul are taken from the publication Pregnancy Care. This is copyright of the NSW Health Department, which has kindly given me permission to use its work in this manual. Thank you Maree Callinan and Debra Lynn.

Jenny Devine has combined her skills at both podiatry and reflexology and contributed a piece on Biomechanics of the Feet in Pregnancy. Thank you Jenny.

A dear multi-skilled friend Farida Irani has contributed information about feet from India. Thank you Farida.

Two reflexologists 'extraordinaire", Anne Thomas and Val Groome have contributed some of their insights. Thank you both.

Melissa Cooney has generously agreed to let me reprint her poignant encounter with pregnant feet. Melissa, thank you.

Lastly a very big Thank you to all participants from my workshops and classes who have taught me so much about a topic that I am passionate about.

THANK YOU EVERYONE
Susanne Enzer

Maternity Reflexology Manual

Part 1: Basics

Part 2: Preconception

Part 3: Pregnancy

Appendices

Indexes

Part 1: Basics

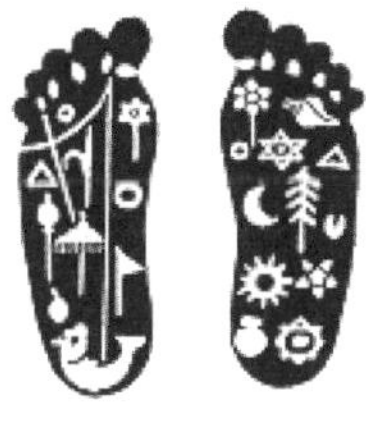

Introduction to Basics

The basics for Maternity Reflexology include:

A sound knowledge

The basics for Maternity Reflexology are a sound knowledge of the bones of both the feet and the female pelvis.

A basic understanding

It is important to have a basic understanding of the anatomy and physiology of the female reproductive system and where it is located on the foot reflex zones.

An interest

To broaden the outlook and for interest sake to wet the appetite for more, a brief look at other aspects of "footy stuff'.

HISTORIC FEET

Part of a definition of reflexology is that it is *"an ancient natural therapy"*. Maternity Reflexology also has its roots in ancient mythology and folklore.

MYTHOLOGY AND FOLKLORE

Masculine aspect

From the masculine aspect mythology and folklore ascribe strength and adventure to the feet.

Feminine aspect

From the feminine aspect the feet are associated with fertility and the sacred female.

Sacred feet

The feet of women are an ancient symbolism found in many parts of the world and are considered sacred. *"The foot established a connection between the life-giving earth and the gods, goddesses, heroines and saints, these deities and persons were credited with possessing healing power which enabled them to heal or strengthen those who won their favour."* (J. Kirkup, The Foot You Never Knew)

Sexy feet

"Woman was supposed to derive her procreative power from contact with the earth, the mother of all things, thus her foot became the symbol of the fecundating principal." (J. Kirkup, The Foot you Never Knew)

Symbol of fecundity

"In many parts of the world the foot, especially the foot of a woman, has been and still is used as a symbol of fecundity. This symbolism is very ancient. By virtue of the fact that the foot established a connection between the fecund and life giving earth and the gods/goddesses. Woman was supposed to derive her procreative power from contact with the earth, the mother of all things, thus her foot became the symbol of the fecundating principle. After a while, the fructifying power was possessed not only by her foot but even by the footprint, the sandals and shoes of goddesses, queens etc.." (Karl Menninger)

The footprint of Isis

The footprint of the Egyptian goddess Isis was said to have the power to make barren women fertile.

THE FEET

Structure
The feet are mobile weight-bearing structures.

Function
The bones with their muscles and tendons are designed for strength, mobility, balance, support, shock absorption and leverage in motion.

Biomechanics
Leonardo da Vinci described the feet as *"a masterpiece of engineering"*. The feet have multiple intricate movements to fulfill the function requirements.
(See Biomechanics of the Feet and Pregnancy, page 172).

Senses
The feet not only have tactile abilities but also incredible proprioceptive qualities.

Metaphysical aspects

Link to earth energies
The feet are concerned with grounding the individual by being a link between the human energies and the earth energies.
As with all the focal points the energies move both ways, for example, earthing / grounding the individual and supporting her with earth energies.

Life path
The feet take a person along their life path, straight and narrow, up hill, down dale, bumpy and smooth.

Movement for change
Feet create the movement for change. Heads think about it, hands handle it and feet do it!

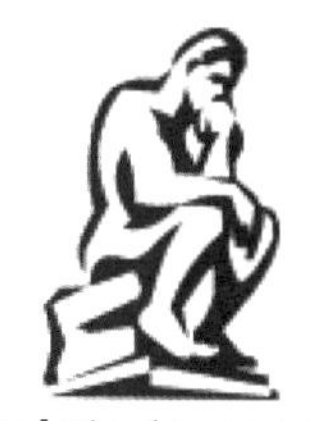

Points to consider

A reflexologist could get insights about the client with:

- Sturdy, broad feet
- Slim feet
- Flat feet
- High longitudinal arch
- Rigid feet
- Supple feet
- Floppy feet
- Different sized feet

What insights occur you?

Bones

THE BONES OF THE FEET

The bones of the feet

Each foot has 26 bones:

- 14 Phalanges (toe bones)
- 5 Metatarsals (long bones)
- 3 Cuneiforms (wedge bones)
- 1 Navicular (boat shaped)
- 1 Cuboid (like a cube)
- 1 Talus
- 1 Calcaneus (heel bone)

LEFT MEDIAL ASPECT

LEFT PLANTAR ASPECT

phalange

metatarso-phalangeal joint (MPJ)

metatarsal 1

cuneiform

navicular

talus

sub-talar joint

calcaneus

LEFT LATERAL ASPECT

LEFT DORSAL ASPECT

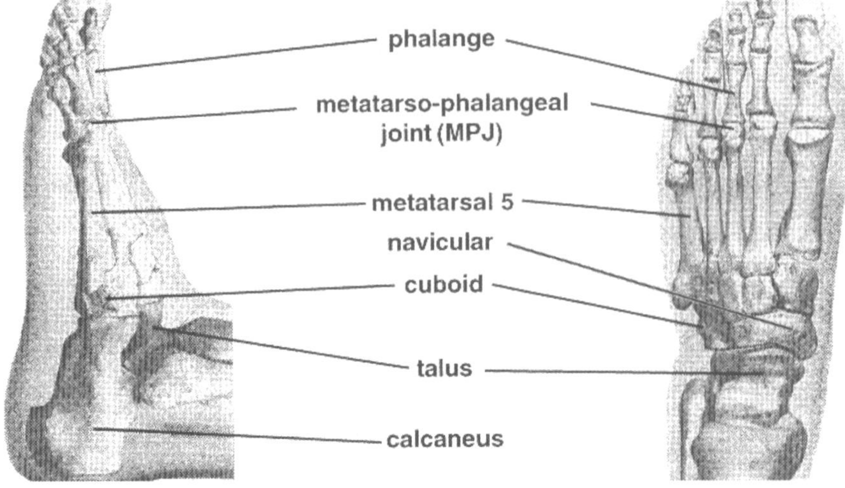

Metaphysical aspects

Principle of Correspondences

According to the Metamorphic Technique modality the skeleton corresponds to the structure and core of our physical being providing a solid inner foundation. Metaphysically it is the skeleton / framework of our life. (Gaston Saint-Pierre)

Weight bearer

Talus is a weight bearer. It bears the weight of the entire body. Energetically it relates to sacrum, which bears the weight of the head and torso and Atlas that bears the weight of the head.

Mother Earth contact

Calcaneus the heel bone is the prime contact with Mother Earth and plays an important part in walking. It is the initial element of gait and as such involved in undertaking movement and change.

Mother Principal

According to the Metamorphic Technique modality the heel holds the Mother Principal (Gaston Saint-Pierre).

Points to consider

A reflexologist could get insights about the client with:

- Painful spur on the heel
- Spur on the navicular
- Broken foot bone(s)

What insights occur to you?

How may the insights enrich the reflexology treatment?

BONES OF THE FEMALE PELVIS

The structure

The structure of the female (gynaecoid) pelvis differs from the male (android) pelvis - it is rounder and wider in all dimensions so that it has the capacity for child bearing and birthing.

The bony pelvis

The bony pelvis (pelvic girdle) is a structure made up of:

Two innominate (coxal) bones. Each innominate bone comprises:

- Ilium (hip bone)
- Ishcium, (sitting bone)
- Pubis (pubic bone)

Sacrum
Coccyx (tail bone)

Two parts

The "false pelvis", the upper part of the pelvis, is basin shaped. It creates a firm structure and does not affect the birthing process.

The "true pelvis" also known as the inner pelvis, is cylindrical shaped and is the bony part of the birth canal. It is of great importance during birthing, as the baby must pass through it.

SIDE OF SKELETON

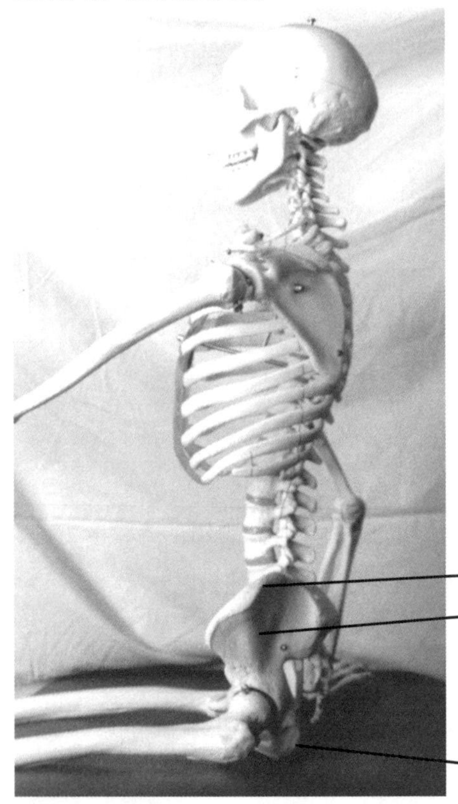

FRONT OF SKELETON

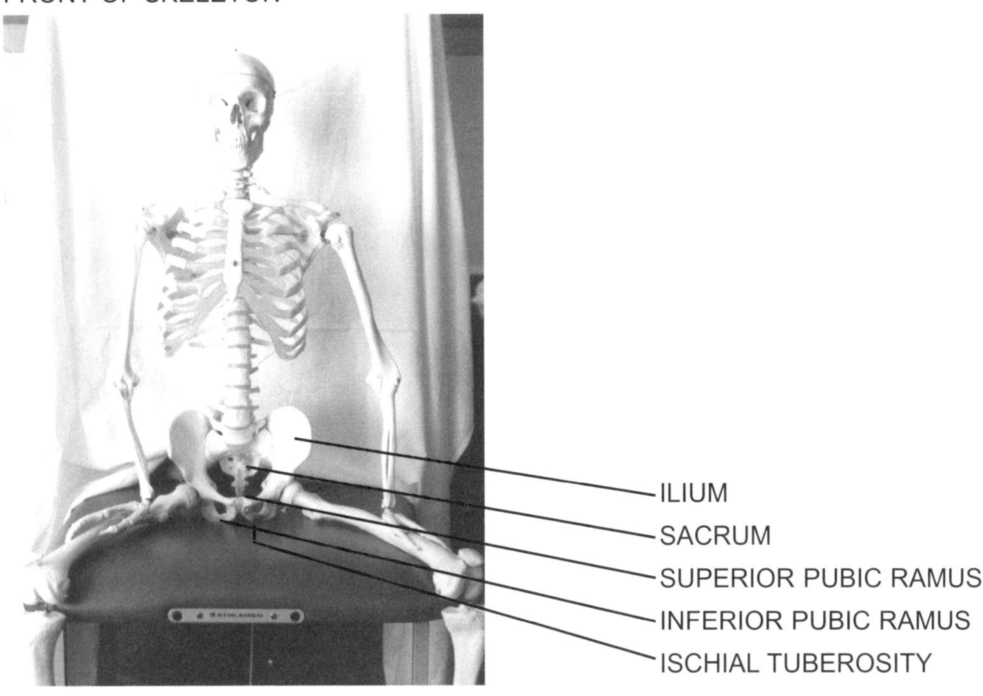

BACK OF SKELETON

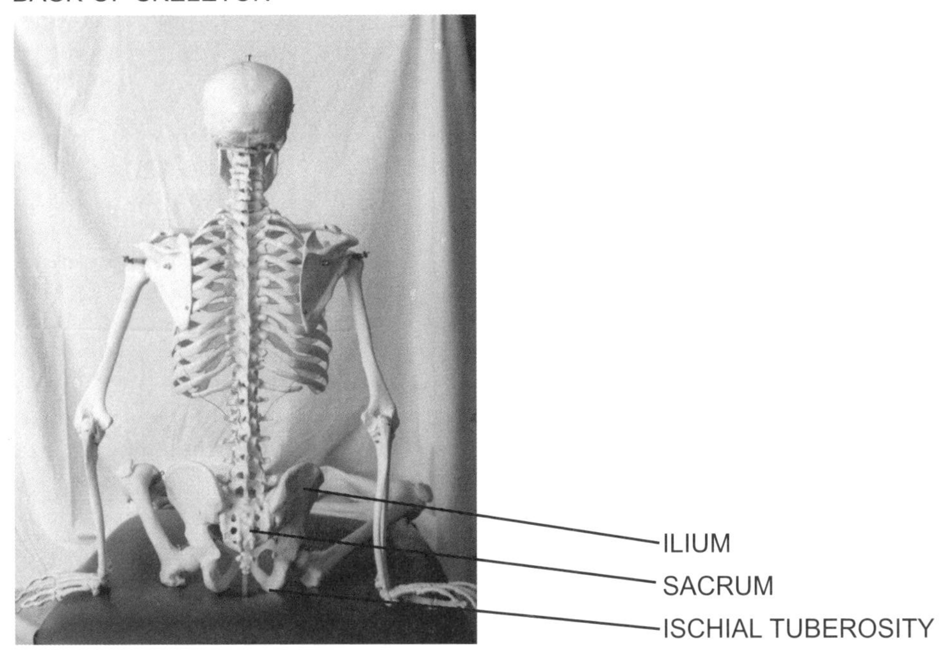

Metaphysical aspects

The female pelvic bones — The female pelvic bones relate to the protection of fertility and the essence of the next generation.

Hips — The hips are the major joint for forward movement and stability.

Sacrum — The sacrum is not only part of the pelvis but also the lower part of the spine. It relates to weight bearing, protection and support, the support being physical support of security.

DIRECT SOMATIC REPLICATION OF THE BONES OF THE PELVIS ON THE BONES OF THE FEET

There is a clear correlation of the shape of the bones of the pelvis and the bones of the feet. In this text it is called "the direct somatic replication".

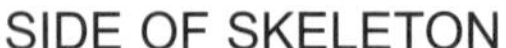

SIDE OF SKELETON

LATERAL ASPECT OF FOOT

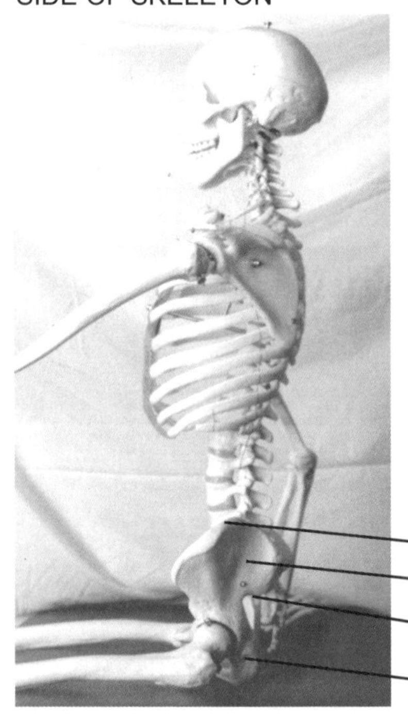

FRONT OF SKELETON

PLANTAR ASPECT OF FEET

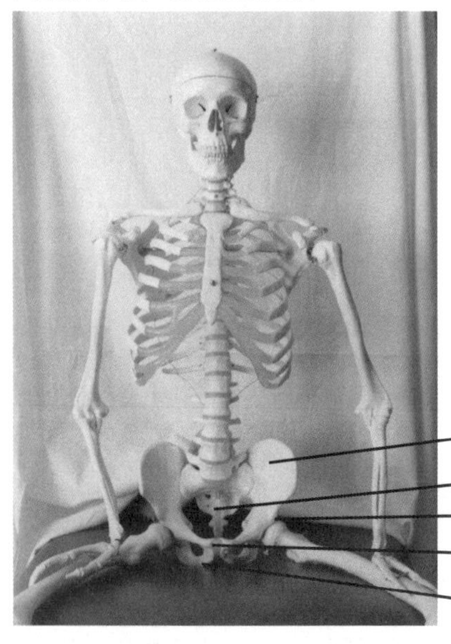

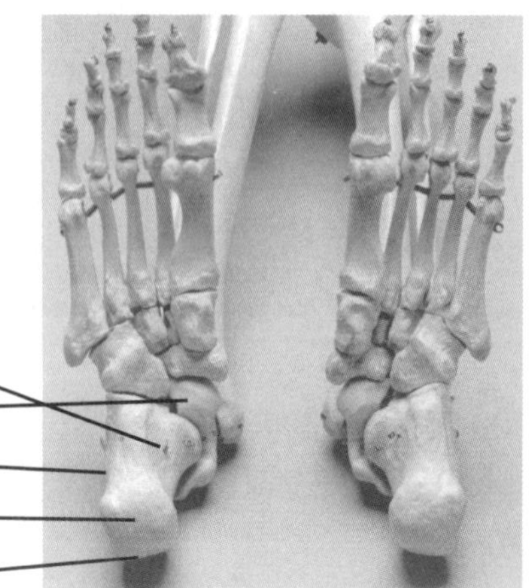

* Anterior Superior Iliac Spine (ASIS)

BACK OF SKELETON

DORSAL ASPECT OF FEET

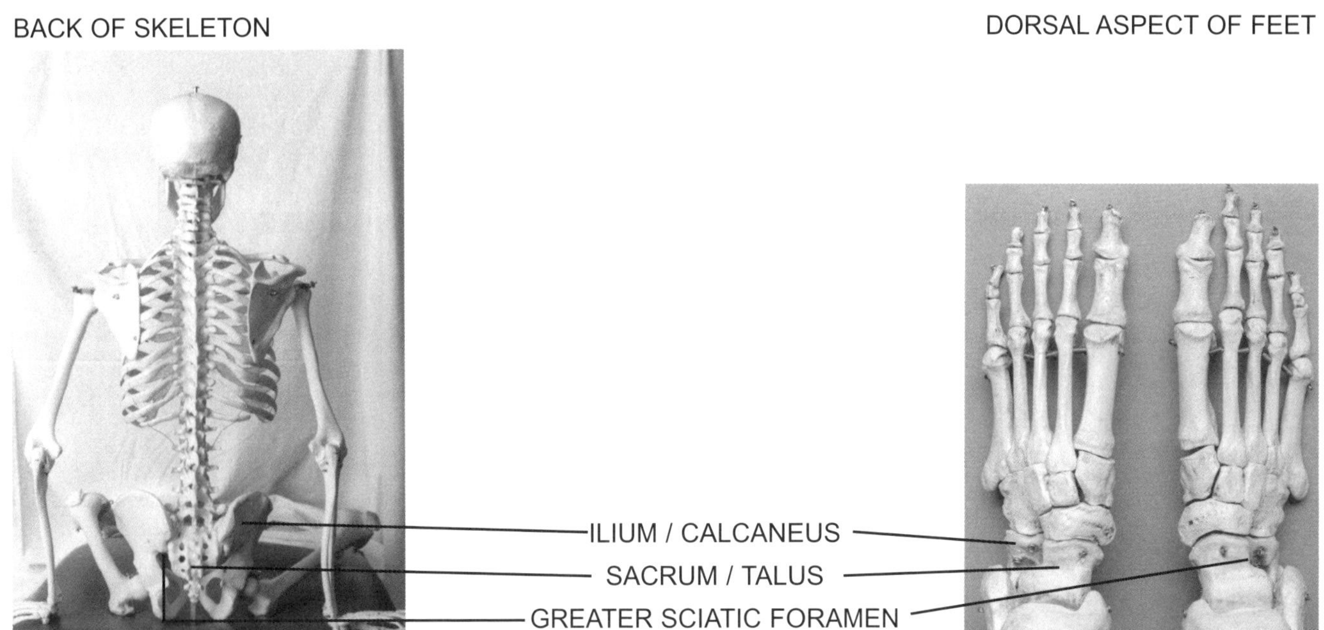

MEDIAN PLANE OF THE SKELETON

In the pelvis, bones crossing the mid-line of the skeleton are sacrum and symphysis pubis. As no photo can be taken of this aspect a diagram is used in this text.

DIAGRAM OF SPINE

LEFT MEDIAL ASPECT

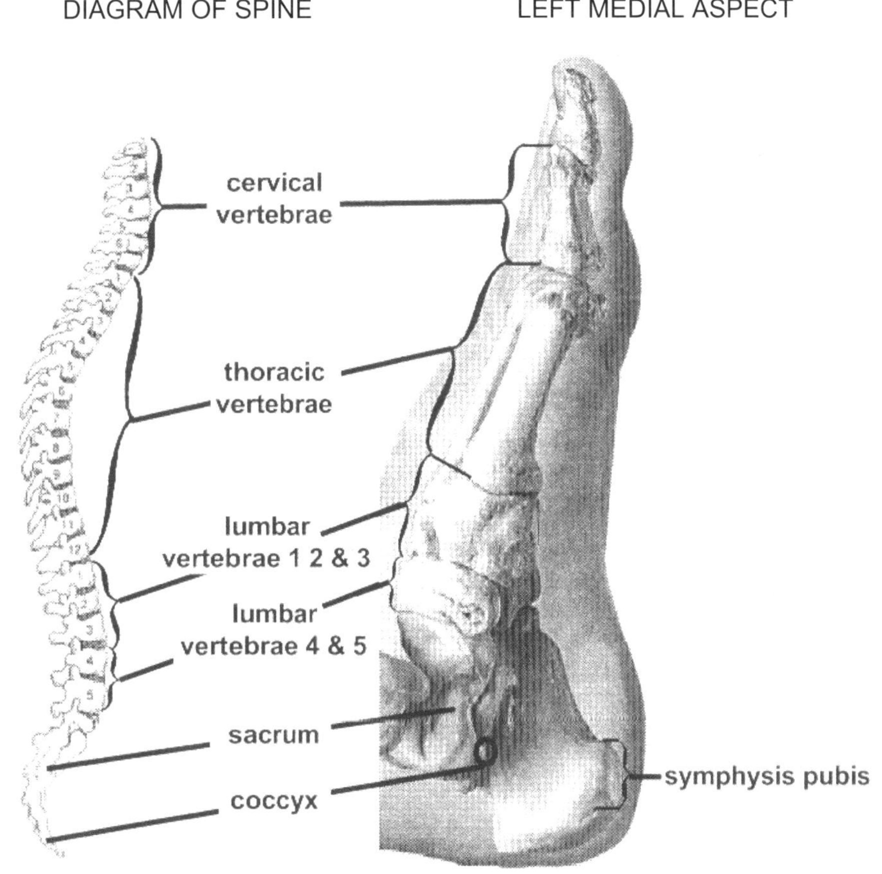

Reflexology Techniques

Reflexologists use many techniques to gain information about their clients.
To gain information about the bony structure requires another technique. In this text it is called "palpation".

REVIEW OF INFORMATION GATHERING TECHNIQUES

OBSERVING

Observing	Observing is a technique that many reflexologists do without realising it!
Watching	Observation includes watching: ● The way the client walks ● The attitude of her feet
Looking	Looking at marks, blemishes, calluses and so on.
Seeing	Seeing what is going on with the client. Seeing and sensing are closely linked.
Metaphysical aspect	Using the Principle of Correspondences with observing will give the reflexologist information about the animation of the client.

FEELING

Touching / feeling	Feeling is the technique probably most used by reflexologists. Thumb and finger walking are the bases of most touch techniques. Feeling gives reflexologists information about the vitality or lack of energy, order or disorder in the reflex zones. A large amount of reflexology therapy is based on this information.
Metaphysical aspect	Using the Principle of Correspondences with feeling will give the reflexologist information about the effects of the client's mind (soft tissue) and her emotions (fluids).

SENSING

Sensing	Sensing is a technique that is surprising when reflexologists first notice that they are using it. Sensing is not so much a physical technique as an "unclear felt sense" that seems to involve the seventh sense. Sensing gives the reflexologist information about things unsaid and unseen. It is especially useful for Maternity Reflexology when sensing the Incoming Soul. It is considered more fully in Part 4, The Incoming Soul & Pregnant Feet.
Metaphysical aspect	Sensing itself is a metaphysical aspect.

PALPATING

Palpating	Palpating is a technique that gives the reflexologist information about structures, both foot structures and direct somatic replication structures.
Metaphysical aspect	Using the Principle of Correspondences with palpating will give the reflexologist information about the basic structure of the client and her life.

PALPATING THE DIRECT SOMATIC REPLICATION OF THE PELVIS ON THE FEET

There are only two bones of the pelvis replicated on two bones of each foot. The innominate bone (large solid bone) is replicated on calcaneus (large solid bone) and sacrum replicated on talus. The trick is to precisely figure out what bit is where.

Method

Instruct the fingers to give information about the bones. Pay no attention to information about reflex zones.

Note

This may be easier said than done for some reflexologists who are used to feeling and sensing.

BOTTOM OF THE PELVIS

Sitting bone
Ischial tuberosity / back of calcaneus

Start with the left foot, use the fingers of the right hand and feel the bone at the back of the heel.
Note the chunkiness of it.

SIDE OF THE PELVIS

Hip bone
Lateral aspect ilium / lateral aspect calcaneus

Move the fingers to the side (lateral aspect) of the heel. This is a large area - use four fingers and have a good feel around.
Note how large it is.

BACK OF THE PELVIS

Sciatic area
Greater sciatic foramen / soft spot on the posterior aspect of talocalcaneal joint

Keeping fingers in touch with bone, crawl the four fingers towards the back (dorsum) of the foot. As the fingers leave the heel bone and the before they reach talus there is a soft spot (replication of the greater sciatic foramen) - be very gentle as this is often painful.

LOWER BACK

Posterior aspect of sacrum / dorsal aspect talus

Although the talus is a large bone most of it is under the end of the leg bones and there is room for only one finger on talus.
Using the length of one finger place it flat on the back (dorsum) of the foot in front of the ankle.

FRONT OF THE PELVIS

Front of pelvis
Iliac crest, ASIS & superior pubic ramus / inferior aspect of calcaneus

When looking at a skeleton the bones of the replication of the front of the pelvis can be seen. However they cannot be palpated on a "lived in" foot.

Symphysis pubis
Symphysis pubis / medial process of calcaneus

Place the tips of two fingers on the medial aspect of the heel bone. It feels like a bony ridge.

Caution

Until confidant to palpate this bone, do not practice this on a first trimester pregnant client.

INNER PELVIS

Inside / back
Sacral curve / sub-talar joint

To locate talus, place a finger on the inner anklebone then slide it down a bit. The bone immediately distal to the leg bones is talus. Using three fingers palpate talus. Once the fingers have located the bone palpate the lower edge of talus - the sub-talar joint.

Note

Maternity Reflexologists frequently use the reflex zone of the symphysis pubis to ease the pain of the condition separated symphysis, and the reflex zone of the sacral curve to promote healing of the sacrum after traumatic delivery.

Organs

ORGANS OF THE FEMALE PELVIS

The location

The organs of the female pelvis are contained within in the true / inner bony pelvis.

Anatomy of the female pelvis

The organs of the female pelvis:

- Bladder and urethra
- Rectum and anus
- Uterus and vagina

Arteries and veins

Pelvic nerves

Pelvic lymphatic system

Principle of Correspondences

According to the Metamorphic Technique modality the soft tissue has a correspondence with the mental aspect (the effects of the mind) and expresses the continual movement of change within us. The pelvic organs are affected by this concept.

Metaphysical aspects
Base chakra

The energies of the Base (first / root) Chakra predominate in the pelvis.
"The first chakra vortex creates matter." (A. Judith)
"The first chakra is associated with primordial life, energy and trust. Relationship to the earth and the material world. Stability and power to achieve." (S. Sharamon)
"The female root chakra rotates to the left, making women more receptive for the stimulating and life-giving power of the earth flowing through the root centre." (S. Sharamon)

BLADDER

Anatomy & physiology

The bladder is part of the urinary tract, which comprises: kidneys, ureters, bladder and urethra. The bladder is a muscular sac that stores and eliminates urine.
It is usually situated in the pelvis behind the pubic bone. A full bladder and at times during pregnancy and during birthing it becomes an abdominal organ.
During pregnancy in the first few weeks the newly gravid uterus squashes the bladder causing frequency of micturition. In the last few weeks the baby's head in the pelvis squashes it again, with the same results.

Associated emotions

Frustration, annoyance, "pissed off". The bladder is also affected by the kidney emotions of fear, terror and dread.

Metaphysical aspects

According to the Principle of Correspondences (Metamorphic Technique) the fluids of the body correlate with fluids in nature and correspond with emotions. In nature fluids such as rain, rivers, sea and so on must keep moving or problems occur. The same applies to the emotions.

RECTUM

Anatomy & physiology

The rectum is the last part of the alimentary tract. It is a muscular tube that stores and eliminates faeces.
It is situated in the pelvis anterior to the sacrum.
During pregnancy progesterone makes the plain muscles relax creating sluggish colon activity. More water is absorbed from the colon making stools harder.
One of the prodromal signs of imminent start to birthing is that the bowel empties.

Associated emotions

Security or the lack of, "the shits".

Metaphysical aspects

According to the Principle of Correspondences (Metamorphic Technique) the effects of the mind are recorded in the soft tissue of the body, which in this case includes the alimentary tract.

UTERUS

Anatomy & physiology

The uterus, vagina, fallopian tubes and ovaries make up the female reproductive system.
The uterus is a specialised muscular organ. It is involved in fertility cycles and sheds its lining (endometrium) each menstruation.
It receives the fertilised ovum, provides a suitable environment for the growth and development of the foetus throughout pregnancy and assists in the expulsion of the baby and placenta at birth.

Before pregnancy the uterus is a small pelvic organ that weighs about 50g. By the end of pregnancy it is a large abdominal organ that weighs about 1,100g. (Mayes' Midwifery) a 2,200% increase in size! To achieve this enormous growth the uterus lays down more muscular tissue and increases its blood supply.

Associated emotions

Ever changing with the cycles of the menstrual cycle and all emotions during the progress of pregnancy.

Metaphysical aspects

The uterus is the organ that holds the qualities of the supreme woman. It is the quintessence of her being.

Points to consider

What insights may the reflexologist get about the client who has:

- Thick, hard, cracked skin around her heels
- Deep groove below the ball of her big toe
- Callused area on the balls of her feet
- Plantar warts on her heels
- Fungal infection between her little toe and fourth toe
- Ankle oedema
- Sweaty feet
- Purple looking veins on her inner ankles
- Thick ankles?

Why would it be advisable NOT to buy new shoes during pregnancy?

After she has had her first baby do the client's pre-pregnancy shoes still fit? Do her feet return to her maiden size?

FOOT REFLEX ZONES OF THE FEMALE ORGANS OF THE PELVIS

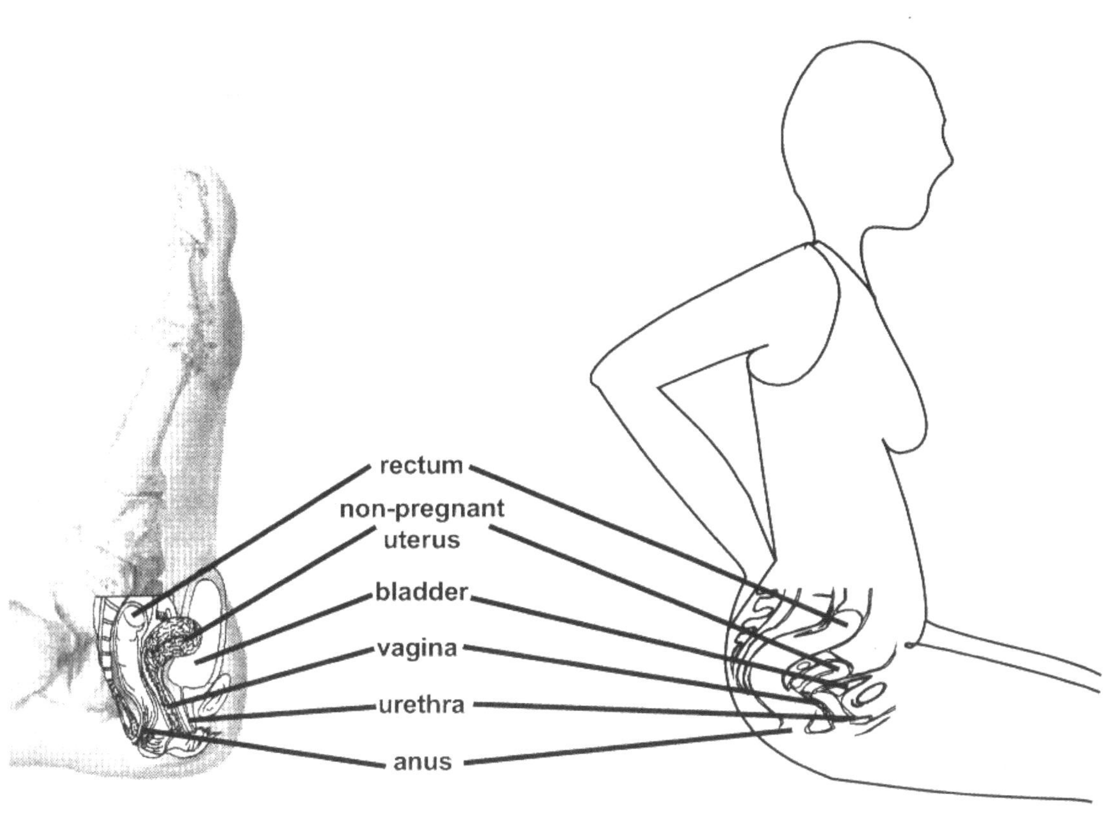

All the areas indicated on the diagram are located on both feet.

Part 2: Preconception

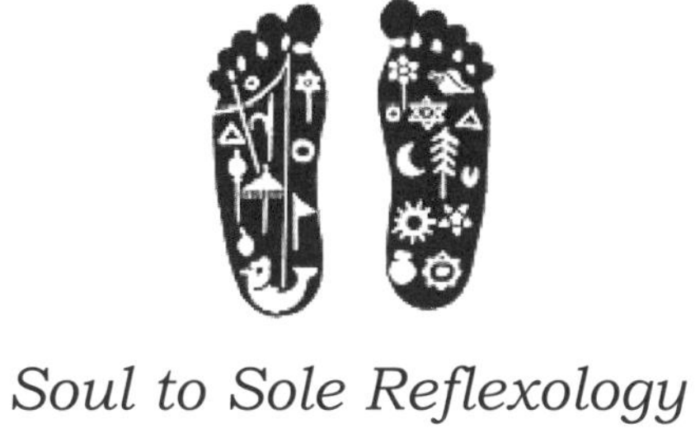

Soul to Sole Reflexology

Introduction To Preconceptual Care

About 90% of conceptions are by mistake! Frequently a happy mistake; however it means that many couples do not receive preconceptual care.

Preconceptual care Preconceptual care is preparing body, mind and spirit for the every-day miracle of conceiving, developing and birthing an Incoming Soul.

Incoming Soul Incoming Soul is a term the author has chosen to use to encompass preconceptual energy, fertilised ovum, group of cells, embryo, foetus and finally the baby.

Important undertaking Creating a person is such an important undertaking, bringing with it enormous changes to everything the couple have already known. So it is very sensible to be as well prepared as possible.

The couple Ideally both partners should be included in preconceptual care. Both sperm and ova need to be healthy. According to Francesca Naish *"the formation of sperm may take up to 116 days and ova are susceptible to damage during their period of maturation...approximately 100 days".*

Recommended reading *"The Natural Way to Better Babies, Preconception Health Care for Prospective Parents",* by Francesca Naish and Jeanette Roberts.

Reflexology Reflexology as a natural therapy that deals holistically with clients is an ideal modality for preconceptual care.

The Fertile Couple

It takes two to tango! With Maternity Reflexology most time will be spent with the woman; however please always remember the man.

MAN'S FERTILITY

The child

The male child already has his hormones of fertility (androgens) but they are not of sufficient quantity to make him fertile.

The adolescent

At about fourteen years of age the boy has a surge in the quantity of his androgens. For several years the levels keep increasing and he becomes fertile.

The man

Once the man has reached his maximum level of androgens he maintains that level for a few years then the levels decrease by 5% per year thereafter.

WOMAN'S FERTILITY

There are three major transitions for a woman during her fertile life:

- from CHILD to MAID via MENARCHE
- from MAID to MOTHER via PREGNANCY
- from MOTHER to MATRIARCH via MENOPAUSE.

The Child

The female child already has her hormones of fertility but they are not of sufficient quantity to make her fertile.

Child to Maid

At about ten to fourteen years of age her fertility hormones escalate, she has several anovulatory cycles.
Menarche is the first menstrual period.

Maid

The natural menstrual cycles for the maid coincide with her lunar cycles and occur thirteen times a year.

Maid to Mother

Pregnancy is the transition from maid to mother and specific-to-pregnancy hormones are produced.
After birthing the hormones of breast-feeding take effect. After that she returns to her fertility cycles.

Mother to Matriarch

This is another transition when the fertility hormones are diminishing. Menopause.

Matriarch

The woman still has her hormones of fertility; however they are not of sufficient quantity to make her fertile.

AN "OVA" VIEW

This diagram gives an impression of menstrual cycles joined together to make a lifetime's menstrual spiral - an "ova view".

MAID MOTHER MATRIARCH

MENARCHE
At ± 12 years

MENOPAUSE
At ± 52 years

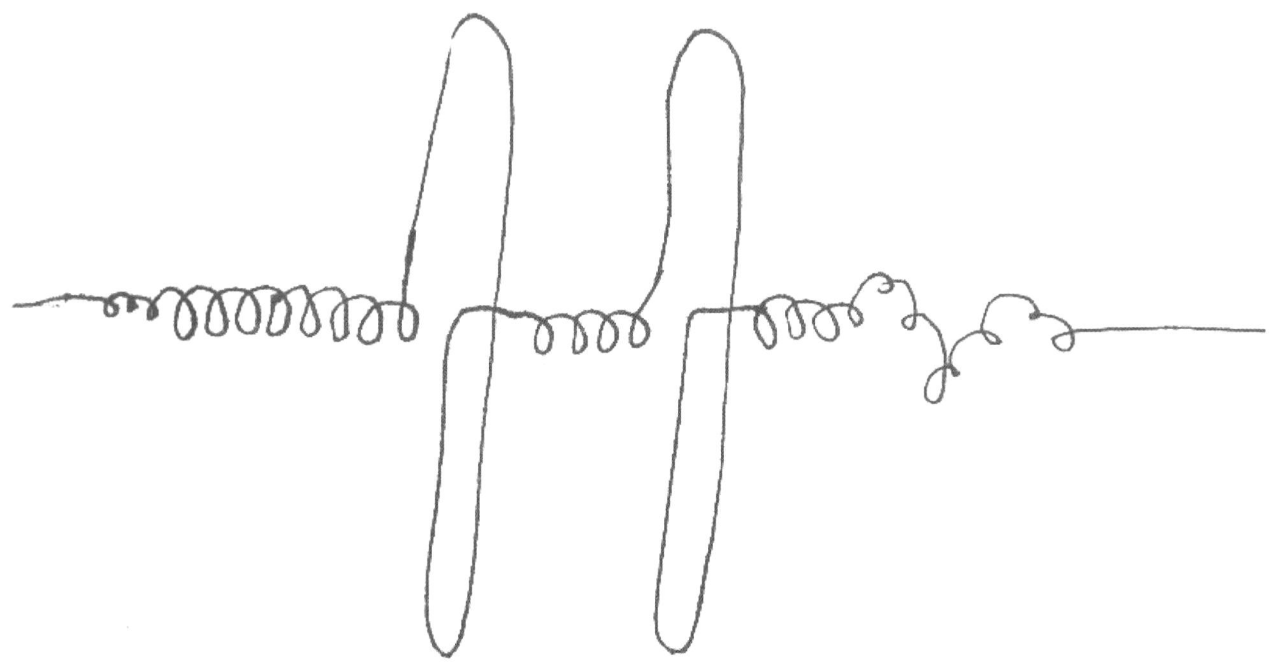

TOTAL YEARS OF FERTILITY
± 40 years

The hormones of fertility and pregnancy play an enormous part in women's lives. To enable the reflexologist to have a "feel" for their female clients the next few pages are devoted to female hormones of fertility.

THE FERTILITY CYCLES

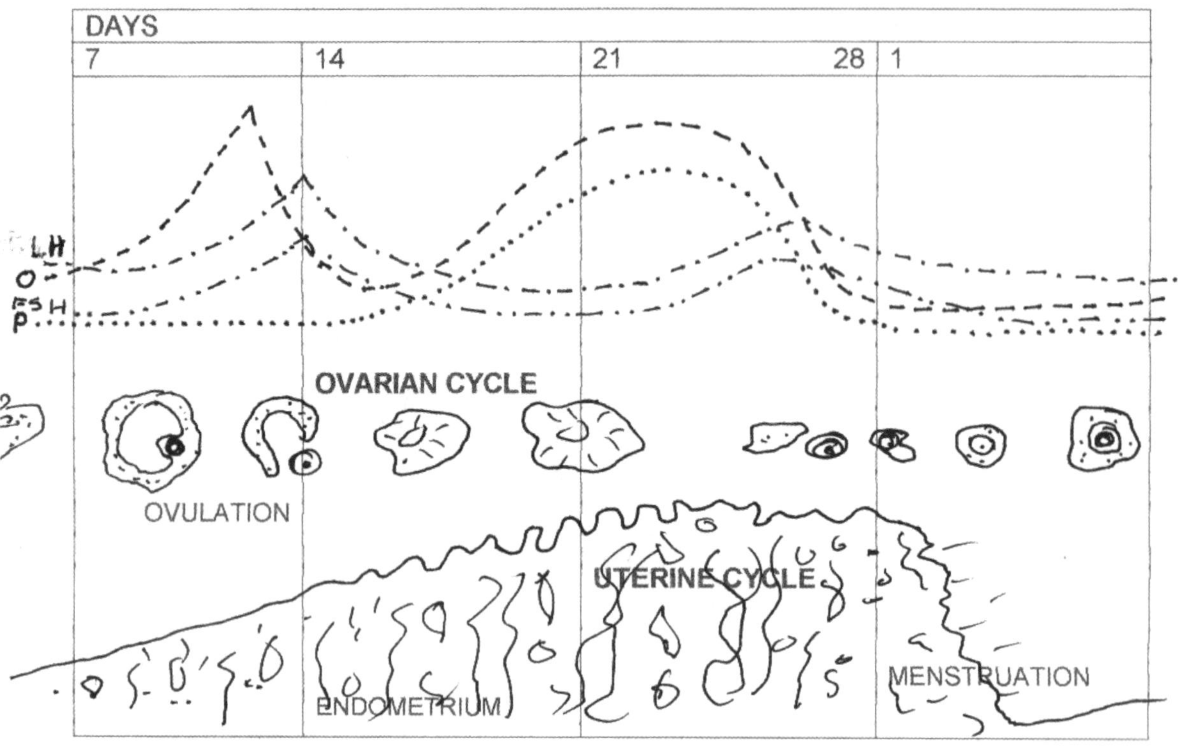

This diagram represents the twenty-eight days of a natural menstrual cycle.

Uterine cycle

The lower part of the diagram shows the uterine cycle. At menstruation the endometrium (lining of the uterus) is shed. Under the influence of hormones it is rebuilt, prepared for an implantation. If no pregnancy occurs it diminishes then is discarded. Menstruation is counted as day one of the cycle.

Ovarian cycle

The middle part of the diagram shows the ovarian cycle. Under the influence of hormones the ovary is prepared, an ovum (egg) develops then ovulation occurs. After ovulation the body of the ovary is maintained and the next follicle is prepared. Ovulation occurs fourteen days before menstruation.

Fertility hormones

The upper part of the diagram shows the fluctuating levels of four fertility hormones.

HORMONES OF FERTILITY

FOUR PRINCIPLE FERTILITY HORMONES

Luteinizing Hormone (LH)

LH is produced in the Pituitary gland.
One of its functions is to create a lipid rich environment in the ovary. There is a surge in the level of LH at ovulation, it then reduces and begins to rise before menstruation.

Follicle Stimulating Hormone (FSH)

FSH is produced in the Pituitary gland.
Its function is to stimulate the ovary to develop a new follicle in preparation for the next ovarian cycle.

Oestrogen

Oestrogen is an ovarian hormone. Two of its functions are to develop and maintain female body characteristics and to be involved in the menstrual cycle.

Progesterone

Progesterone is an ovarian hormone that prepares the uterus for pregnancy and is involved in the menstrual cycle.

The above is a very brief description of the fertility hormones.

Suggested further study

- Gonad Releasing Hormone (GnRH).
- Follicle Stimulating Hormone (FSH).
- Luteinizing Hormone (LH).
- Oestrogen.
- Progesterone.

THE EFFECTS OF THE HORMONES OF FERTILITY

The hormones of fertility and pregnancy have a profound effect not only on women but also their men-folk, family, colleagues and even strangers.

Recommended resource Video *"The Hormone Hat"* by Grannie-Su Enterprises.

Throughout the forty years of a woman's fertile life she is continually undergoing physical and emotional changes.

The following tables show in order of occurrence the physical changes and some of the emotions that accompany these changes.

CHILD TO MAID

Menarche is the first menstrual period. It occurs during puberty at about 10 to 13 years of age. Puberty is brought about by increased amounts of the hormones of fertility.

PHYSICAL RESPONSE	FEELINGS & EMOTIONS
Child; infertile	Innocent
Fertility hormones increasing	Cheeky, saucy
Increase in fat, change of body shape; breast buds, waist, hips	Pleased, sulky, awkward, teary
Growth of body hair; axillary, pubic	Shy, embarrassed
First period, menarche	Horrified, pleased, proud

MAID

The first part of woman's cycle is from the end of menstruation to ovulation.
This is a time of enticement behaviour.

PHYSICAL RESPONSE	FEELINGS & EMOTIONS
Increased blood flow to the brain, causing clear mind, enhanced verbal skills, acute hearing, clear articulation	Sociable, lively, happy, smiley
Pupils dilate causing more blinking and improved vision	Wide eyed and wonderful, flirtatious
Increased pheromone output. Acute sense of smell - 10,000 times more sensitive to male pheromones	Attractive, gorgeous
Breast changes: proliferation of mammary tissue	Saucy
Erectile tissue (nipples) sensitised	Excited
Cervical mucus changes: increased amount, alkaline, texture, 1 drop stretches 8-12cm (spinbarkeit). Promotes transport of sperm	Lush Sperm friendly fanny!
Basal body temperature rises	Randy, scarlet woman, "tickles the fancy"
Increased libido	Red hot lover
Ovulation	Party time!
Body pauses to give time for sperm (if any) to arrive at the ovum	Content, satisfied

MAID

The second part of woman's cycle is from after ovulation to menstruation.
This is a time of preparation and protection.

PHYSICAL RESPONSE	FEELINGS & EMOTIONS
Cessation of enticement behaviour, prepare for possible pregnancy	Oh dear
Fluid and salt retention, oedema, weight gain, constipation, headache	Bloated, unlovely, "big splot"
Increased blood supply to endometrium, decreased blood supply from head	Silly, incapable, confused, mood swings
Breast changes: lumpy, tender / painful	Lonely, unloving, yearning, prickly
Cervical mucous changes texture to a thick paste. It becomes acidic and hostile to sperm	Hostile, angry, aggressive, unlovable
Blood sugar levels drop. Cold. Carbohydrate craving	Frigid, greedy, unsatisfied, selfish, tired, exhausted
Sebaceous glands produce more sebum - acne, zits	Really ugly, boring, dull, low self esteem
Endometrium becomes ischaemic, is destroyed and prepares to be shed. Pelvic pain, cramps	Dissatisfied, unfulfilled, unsupported, depressed. Need solitude & stillness, Tired, spacey, inward looking
PMT, an excessive, disordered, debilitating, concurrent symptoms	Irritable, tense, fatigued, depressed, maybe suicidal thoughts.
Uterus contracts and sheds the endometrium. Menstruation	Whew! Relief from tension, pride in womanliness, relieved not to be pregnant. Disappointment, sadness, grief at no pregnancy
Return of blood supply to head. Clear minded	Care free, cool, calm, creative

The cycles repeat until conception. The hormones of pregnancy are to be found in Part 3, Pregnancy.

MOTHER TO MATRIARCH

MENOPAUSE

Menopause is the cessation of menstrual periods and is commonly the name used for the phase leading up to menopause. It is the time of transition from Mother to Matriarch and usually begins at about 45 years to 55 years of age. It is brought about by the reduction of fertile ova then the absence of ova. It is dominated by the gradual lessening of the fertility hormones.

PHYSICAL RESPONSE	FEELINGS & EMOTIONS
Irregular periods, weight gain	Drab, chaotic, misunderstood, moody
Breast changes: tender, fatty deposits instead of mammary tissue	Lost the stuffing, sensuousness and nurturing, lonely
Labile temperature control, hot flushes	Wet rag, hot and bothered
No ova left	Lost the lot
Dry vagina	Lost libido, distressed
Increase in facial hair	Worry, panicky
Collagen tissue looses tone	Dried up old whatzit
Pubic and axillary hair goes grey and starts to fall out	Surprised

MATRIARCH

She has had a lifetime of great and ghastly experiences and has acquired the knowledge, wisdom and skills to handle them all.

PHYSICAL RESPONSE	FEELINGS & EMOTIONS
Cessation of menstrual cycles. Infertile	Complete. Can now live in her own true colours. Fantastic

Reflexology Techniques

THE REFLEXOLOGY ENDOCRINE BALANCE

CONCEPTS

Menstrual cycles	As women live through their menstrual cycles the hormones of fertility are changing all the time. No two cycles are the same - each one is in a different month, a different season and different year. The cycles are also affected by everything else that is happening in the woman's life: her diet, exercise, home and work, relationships and so on.
Useful reflexology technique	The reflexology endocrine balance is a very useful reflexology technique to balance the woman to wherever she is in her cycle.
Endocrine glands - a unit	Although the endocrine glands are to be found in different places about the body, they work as a unit and support and complement each other.
Balance	The reflexology endocrine balance therefore balances the entire system.
Concepts of reflexology	This technique uses holistic concepts of reflexology to balance body, mind and spirit.
Physical	The physical body is reflected in the feet - the direct somatic reflexion.
- Access to physical energies	To access the physical energies use firm pressure for treatment or relaxation techniques.
Emotions and feelings	The emotions and feelings are recorded in the feet in the soft tissue as lines, hard skin etc, in the fluids as dry or sweaty feet, oedema etc. and the attitude of the feet.
- Access to emotions and feelings	To access the emotions and feelings use a very light touch for treatment or relaxation techniques.
Etheric energies	The etheric energies are always around; although they are usually invisible, sometimes they may be seen as colours.
- Access to the etheric energies	To access the subtle energies, which are not of a physical nature, use sensing techniques and be open to intuition.
The O-zone	Reflexology uses the concept of ten longitudinal zones along which the reflexology impulses pass. A perception of many reflexologists is that the energy also moves across the space between the feet - the interface between left and right. In this text the space is termed the O-zone. **Note:** Many reflexologists have found that the O-zone has much information of / from the Incoming Soul.

The reflexology endocrine balance uses all the above concepts. It begins by physically stimulating the reflex zones, then uses a light touch to inform the senses that the system is working together. It continues by using the O-zone to balance left and right sides and finishes with intention from the practitioner for balance and harmony.

THE ENDOCRINE GLANDS, ANATOMICAL PLACEMENTS AND REFLEX ZONES

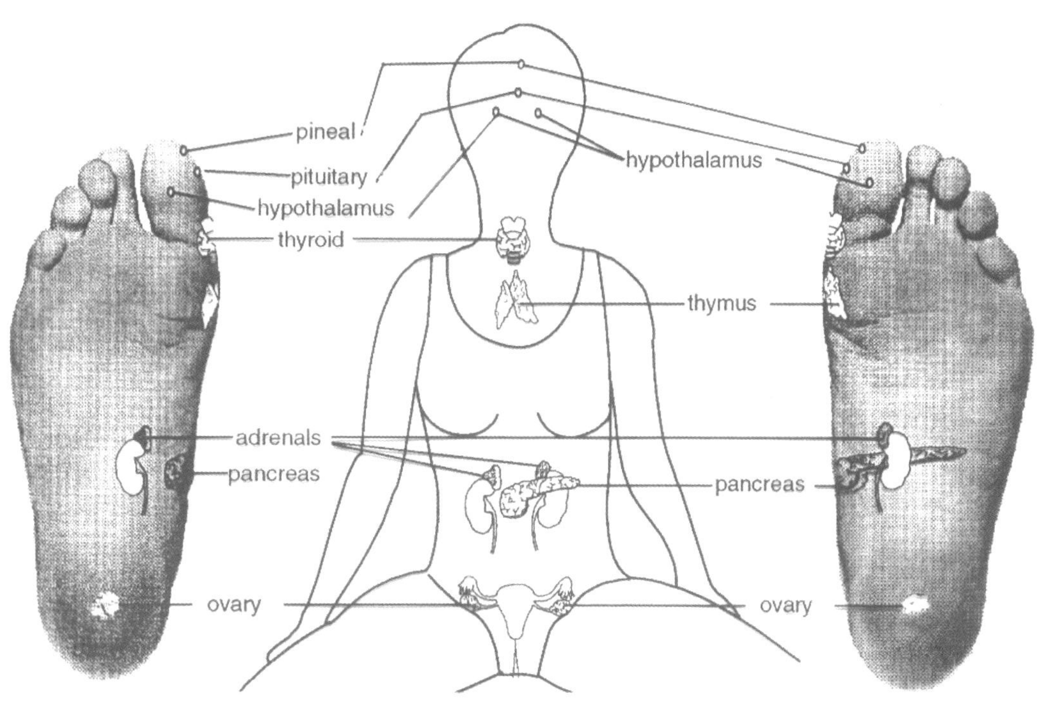

Direct somatic reflexion

The direct somatic reflexion is used in the diagram and may differ from other reflexology charts.

Indirect ovary reflex zone

The frequently used reflex zone for the ovaries, located on the lateral aspect of the heels half way between outer anklebone and the bottom of the heel is not a reflexology direct somatic reflexion. It is an acupressure point Bladder 62. In this text it is termed "indirect ovary reflex zone".

Metaphysical aspect
The Chakra / Endocrine connection

According to Hindu tradition the spiritual energy of the person enters the body through energy vortices known as chakras. That spiritual energy is converted into physical energy (hormones) by the endocrine glands. This is an extremely simplified statement and the reader is recommended to further study the chakras and the endocrine system.

THE ROUTINE

Method

Identify the endocrine system reflex zones.
Work with one hand on each foot simultaneously

1. Stimulate

Begin by stimulating all the endocrine glands.

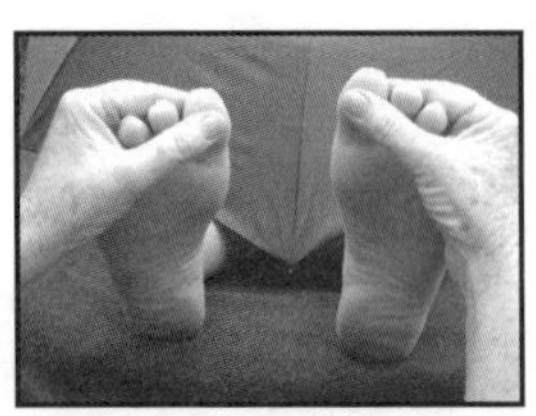

HYPOTHALAMUS

Use the pads of the thumbs.
Press firmly but gently into the reflex zones, withdraw the thumbs about 1mm, bounce gently on the reflex zones.

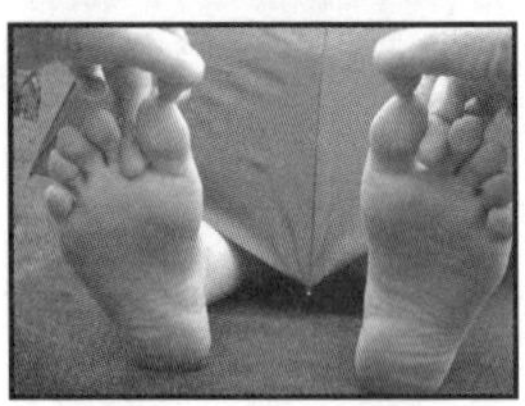

PINEAL

Use the "thumb walking" area of the thumb, thumb walk on the spot.

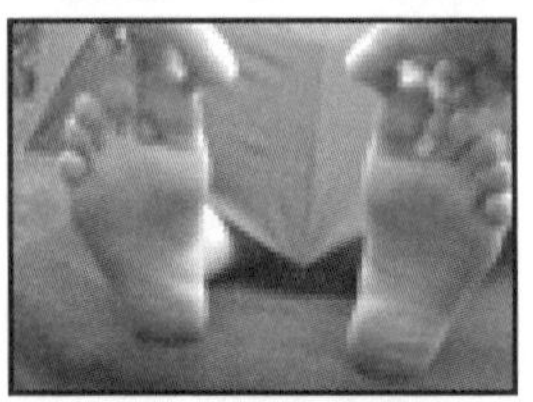

PITUITARY

Use the "thumb walking" area of the thumb, thumb walk on the spot.

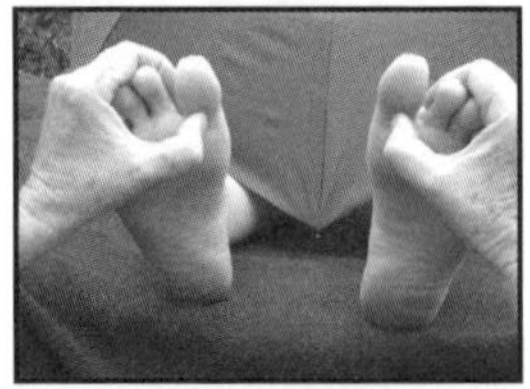

THYROID

"Thumb walk" over the reflex zones.
It is easier from lateral to medial.

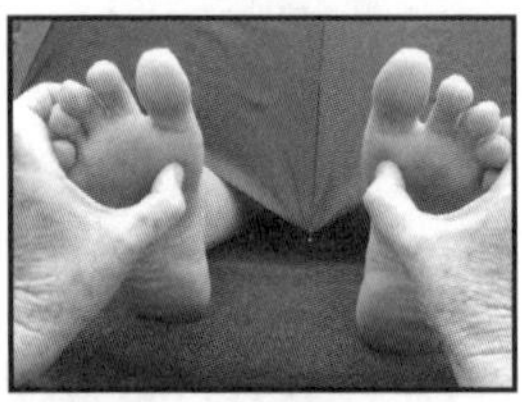

THYMUS

"Thumb walk" and tap the reflex zones.

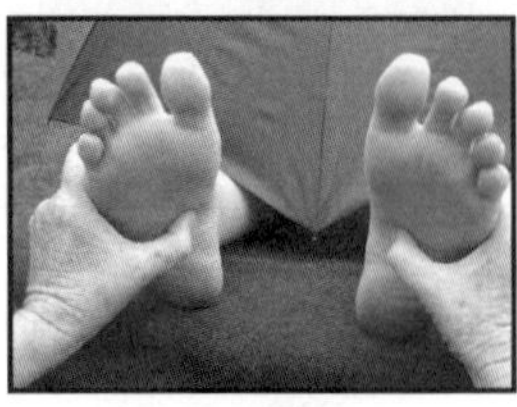

PANCREAS

"Thumb walk" the reflex zones - lateral to medial is easier.

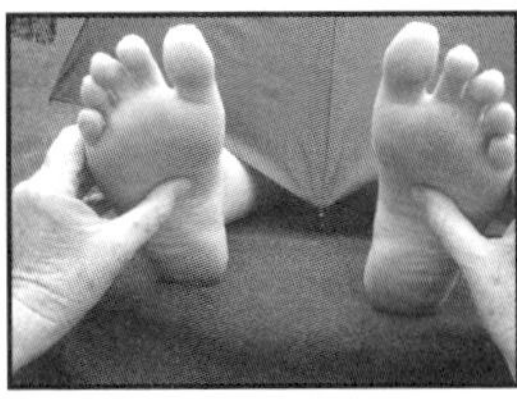

ADRENAL GLANDS

Use the pads of the thumbs, press firmly but gently onto the zones, withdraw about 1mm and bounce gently on the reflex zones. Remember this is the stress gland - be gentle with it.

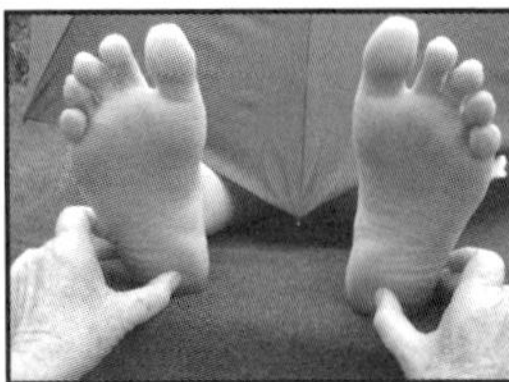

OVARIES

Place the thumbs on the direct ovary reflex zones and your third finger on the indirect ovary reflex zones. Make a pinch like movement.

2. Connect

Now that all the endocrine glands reflex zones are stimulated they are ready for action.

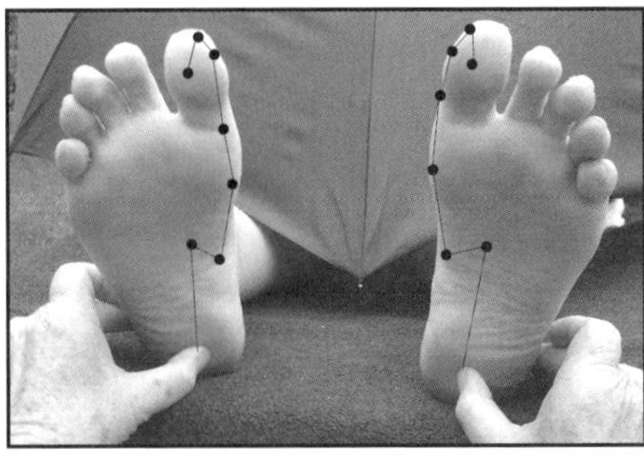

Connect them together to acknowledge that they are a unit. The connecting movement is like a firm stroking movement.

Connect reflex zones of:

- Ovaries to pancreas
- Pancreas to adrenal glands
- Adrenal glands to thymus
- Thymus to thyroid
- Thyroid to pituitary
- Pituitary to pineal and
- Pineal to hypothalamus

3. O-Zone

The next part connects the energies across the O-zone.

Repeat the sequence using a very light touch.

Sense the energy under you fingers set your intention to balance across the O-zone.

If the energy feels the same hold for several seconds and move on to the next zones in the sequence.

If the energies do not feel the same maintain the hold and the intention until you feel a balance or for up to two minutes.

If after two minutes the energy is still not balanced, complete the endocrine balance routine and return to the disordered endocrine gland and if it is appropriate use reflexology therapy to normalise it.

4. Connect

Repeat the connecting stroke.

Connect reflex zones of:

- Ovaries to pancreas
- Pancreas to adrenal glands
- Adrenalglands to thymus
- Thymus to thyroid
- Thyroid to pituitary
- Pituitary to pineal and
- Pineal to hypothalamus

Reflexology Therapy

REFLEXOLOGY

Natural therapy	One of the great strengths of reflexology is that it is a natural therapy; it is not a medical treatment. Many of the disharmonies and disorders that may occur during a woman's fertile life respond well to reflexology therapy.

MENSTRUAL CYCLES

NORMAL MENSTRUAL CYCLE

A well-balanced cycle repeats every 29 to 32 days. Ovulation occurs 14 days before menstruation.

Menstruation lasts 3 to 5 days, has a moderate flow and has a distinctive physical sensation.

Physiology	See previous pages.
Reflexology	Give full reflexology sessions to maintain regular cycles. Adapt the treatment according to where the client is in her menstrual cycle, for example, stimulating before ovulation and gentle and caring before menstruation. Balance any disordered reflex zones.
Be aware	Be aware of the client's menstrual cycle to enable immediate change of treatment if she becomes pregnant.
Metaphysical aspect	The essence of being "Woman".
Recommended reading	*The Lunar Cycle, A Guide to Natural Fertility Control,* by Francesca Naish, 1989

SOME PROBLEMS

IRREGULAR PERIODS

If menstrual periods do not comply with the above stated criteria, they are considered irregular.

Reflexology	Full reflexology sessions. Balance any disordered reflex zones.
Metaphysical aspect	Fluctuating acceptance of womanhood.
Caution 	The client's periods may become more irregular before they settle into a balanced pattern.

DYSMENORRHOEA

Dysmenorrhoea is painful menstrual periods.

Physiology	Contraction and cramping of the uterine muscle.
Reflexology First Aid	Non-pregnant uterus reflex zone, bimanual trigger point release, to relieve the pain and release trapped energy. Hips and pelvis relaxation techniques, to decrease the tension.
Follow-up	This is a first aid remedy and will not get to the root of the problem. Suggest the client has several reflexology sessions.
Metaphysical aspect	*"An imbalance within the feminine force. Possible damage by past traumas especially where there were issues around respect."* (Christine Page)

MENORRHAGIA

Menorrhagia is heavy / excessive menstrual flow.

Reflexology	Full reflexology sessions. Balance any disordered reflex zones.
Metaphysical aspect	*"Tears of frustration, as the feminine part of the individual is denied its creative expression."* (Christine Page)

OLIGOMENORRHOEA

Oligomenorrhoea is scanty menstrual flow.

Reflexology	Full reflexology sessions. Balance any disordered reflex zones.
Metaphysical aspect	A scant commitment to womanliness.

AMENORRHOEA

Amenorrhoea is the absence of menstrual periods. This is natural in young and old females and during pregnancy. If it occurs during a woman's fertile life it is a problem.

Reflexology	Full reflexology sessions. Balance any disordered reflex zones.
Metaphysical aspect	*"A disconnection of the feminine side as it was not acceptable within the world in which they lived."* (Christine Page)

Points to consider

It is possible that doing a natural therapy such as reflexology the client's cycles will settle to her own natural rhythm - her lunar cycle?

PREMENSTRUAL TENSION / SYNDROME

Premenstrual tension / syndrome is excessive, disordered, debilitating, concurrent symptoms occurring befor menstruation.

Reflexology	Give full reflexology sessions and balance any disordered reflex zones. Include linking technique of "sense of self" to heart reflex zone.
Metaphysical aspect	Rejection of the female process. Fear of accepting being "all woman". Allowing confusion to reign. Giving power to outside influences. No time to nurture and honour the female self.

MENOPAUSE

Menopause is the cessation of menstrual periods. For most women it is a natural occurrence and is of no particular problem. However for some women it is an unpleasant experience that can make them feel ill.

Reflexology	Give full reflexology sessions and balance any disordered reflex zones. Include linking technique of "sense of self" to heart reflex zone. A clue to treatment is that whatever problem occurred at the othe times of transition (puberty and pregnancy) will reappear at this t time unless it has already been resolved.
Metaphysical aspect	A deep-seated fear of no longer being wanted, useful or necessa There may be a loathing of the body's aging and fear of being ne death than ever before.
Note	Menopause is included in this text as it is the natural conclusion woman's fertile life and many reflexologists have clients who are experiencing menopause.

Preconceptual Care

GENERAL CARE

When a couple are planning to have a baby it is sensible for both of them to first get in good shape, not only physically but also mentally and spiritually - there will be many unplanned surprises along the way.

So be prepared!

Recommended reading	*The Natural Way to Better Babies,* by Francesca Naish and Janette Roberts, 1996

For a planned pregnancy this is a beautiful time for the couple. They can "make love" not "have sex" and do not have to worry about contraception.

Reflexology	Give full reflexology sessions to attain and maintain health and wellbeing. Balance any disordered reflex zones.
Metaphysical aspect	Some clairvoyants can see an Incoming Soul about the woman for up to two years before it manifests physically and she conceives. Some people are aware of the miracle that is about to happen.
Caution	Be sure to know where the client is in her menstrual cycle because as soon as she conceives reflexology needs to be done very gently.
Note	Where possible "do" reflexology for both the man and woman of the couple.

SOME PROBLEMS

THE SUB-FERTILE COUPLE

Sub-fertility can occur in both men and women and is an in-between state when they are neither infertile nor can yet conceive.

Emotionally

Some women can have problems conceiving as they have had traumatic experiences, such as termination of pregnancy, previous pregnancy and childbirth, fears of unknown origin or are trying too hard to conceive.

Physically

There are many reasons for sub-fertility including, stress, life style, and physical state of health.
For some couples there seems to be no reason at all.

Reflexology

Reflexology already has an excellent reputation with helping sub-fertile couples to conceive. The qualities of reflexology for creating a balanced mind, body and spirit give the best environment for an Incoming Soul. Give full reflexology sessions and balance any disordered reflex zones.

ASSISTED CONCEPTION

Assisted conception is any method of conceiving other than by sexual intercourse. There are several types of assisted conception. In Vitro Fertilisation (IVF) is probably the most well known method.

Emotionally

This client may be distressed by her lack of being able to conceive. She may become so preoccupied with trying to conceive that she cannot think of anything else.

Physically

The IVF program creates a change in the woman's physical environment to enable the production of several ova. It can be physically exhausting. And it is very expensive.

Reflexology

As this client is under medical supervision the reflexologist must have the permission of the specialist to do reflexology.
The balancing, calming qualities of reflexology help enormously to compliment the medical procedures.
Give full reflexology sessions.

Note

In the UK some fertility clinics employ reflexologists.

Contraindication

When the couple is undergoing the IVF program and the woman is taking Clomid or some fertility drug **OMIT** reflexology until her course of drugs is completed.

The rationale

The rationale is that the drugs will make the body produce several ova. A natural therapy such as reflexology will balance the body to produce a single ovum each month and so is not complimentary to the drug regime.

Part 3: Pregnancy

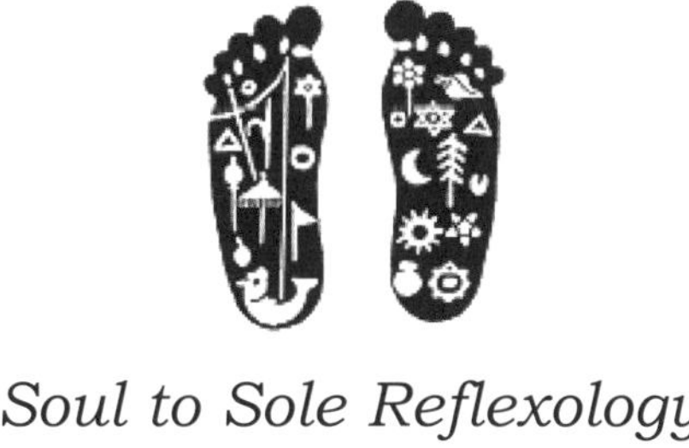

Soul to Sole Reflexology

Introduction to Pregnancy Care

It was once a dream of a politician that all babies should be born equal. A pretty dream but not at all possible as all babies are not even conceived equal. Conception can occur from a multitude of pairings: from a contented couple planning a family to rape, drunken / drugged states, from a very precious long awaited pregnancy or assisted conception to a "one night stand".

Pregnancy care

Pregnancy care is designed to holistically support the client as she evolves through an enormous experience.

Incoming Soul

The Incoming Soul dominates the entire pregnancy. (See Part 4, The Incoming Soul & Pregnant Feet.)

The father

The father has added not only his genes but also his pedigree to the Incoming Soul. This is a time of great changes for the dad.

The mother

For the mother having her first baby it is a major life transition from Maid to Mother.

From the moment of conception (for some women before that moment) huge changes in the being are the norm. Mind, body and spirit are all involved.

With an Incoming Soul manifesting physically within her the woman's sensitivity and intuitiveness are on "high voltage".

Under the influence of the hormones of pregnancy and the developing life within her the woman undergoes enormous physical changes. (These changes are reviewed later.)

Reflexology

A modality such as reflexology is excellent to maintain a balance during the rapidly changing balance of pregnancy.The skill of the reflexologist is to balance and harmonise the whole being. To optimise her health potential. Many of the minor ailments of pregnancy respond well to reflexology therapy. It is important to work within one's own ability and to know when the specialised skills of the obstetric caregiver are needed.

Caution

The complications and disorders of pregnancy **MUST** have expert medical attention.

The Hormones of Pregnancy

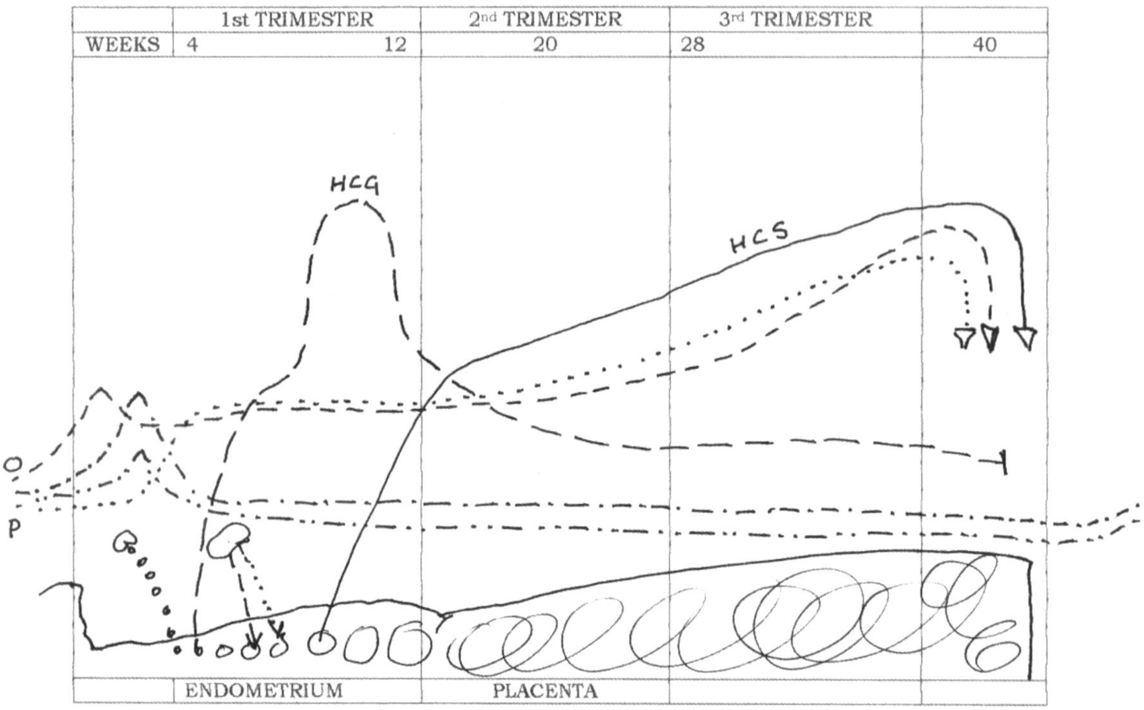

Hormones direct the entire pregnancy. This diagram represents the 40 weeks of pregnancy.

Endometrium / placenta

The lower part of the diagram shows the endometrium and the growing placenta.

Placenta

At implantation the placenta begins to develop, it continues to grow throughout pregnancy.
"The placenta is a complex organ capable of fulfilling all the requirements of the fetus (sic) in utero." (Mayes' Midwifery)

Its functions are:

- Respiratory - a respiratory type function where it enables gas exchange, i.e. oxygen and carbon dioxide.
- Nutritive - it is the vital connection in the transport of vital nutrients.
- Excretory - waste products from the foetus are filtered out.
- Protective - the placental barrier prevents most harmful substances reaching the foetus.
- Hormonal - the placenta produces many hormones which is a fascinating topic to study and will be very simplified in this text.

Pregnancy hormones

The upper part of the diagram shows the increasing levels of hormones throughout pregnancy.

HORMONES OF PREGNANCY

Follicle Stimulating Hormone (FSH) and Luteinizing Hormone (LH)	Neither of these hormones are needed during pregnancy and the. levels remain low.
Oestrogen and Progesterone	Some Oestrogen and Progesterone continues to be produced in the ovary and the placenta produces the greater part.
Human Chorionic Gonadotrophin (HCG)	Human Chorionic Gonadotrophin (HCG) is a hormone produced by the embryo. Its presence in the woman's urine is used as a positive pregnancy test. To implant well and maintain the pregnancy the embryo needs his own special hormone until the placenta is established and able to maintain the pregnancy.
Human Chorionic Somatomammotropin (HCS)	HCS is a placental hormone that is secreted in increasing amounts into the maternal blood. It has similar properties to Human Placental Lactogen, which are involved with growth and metabolism.

Pregnancy Trimesters

Pregnancy is the state of being "with child".

The duration of pregnancy is 40 weeks and is calculated from the first day of the woman's last menstrual period.

THE FIRST TRIMESTER OF PREGNANCY

The first trimester of pregnancy is the first three months or from conception to the end of the twelfth week.

Vital importance	The first trimester of pregnancy is of vital importance for both the Incoming Soul and the mother.
The Incoming Soul	The Incoming Soul has a physical existence. Ensuring his survival he dominates the entire pregnancy. The embryo becomes a foetus and works his way along his own pre-natal pattern. (See Part 4, The Incoming Soul & Pregnant Feet.)
The mother	The mother in the mean time may have many conflicting feelings and emotions ranging from feeling that she has made the biggest mistake in her life to feeling very blessed.
The hormones	Human Chorionic Gonadotrophin (HCG) is a hormone produced by the embryo. Its presence in the woman's urine is used as a positive pregnancy test. To implant well and maintain the pregnancy the embryo needs his own special hormone until the placenta is established and able to maintain the pregnancy. The effects of HCG can create turmoil in the woman; she can feel sick and tired. The effects can last until the pregnancy is well established, that is at about twelve weeks.
Reflexology	During the first trimester of pregnancy all reflexology therapy techniques and relaxation techniques must be done very gently. Observe the precautions and use techniques for general well being.

THE SECOND TRIMESTER OF PREGNANCY

The second trimester is mid-pregnancy - the forth, fifth and sixth months or from week 13 to week 27.

The Incoming Soul The Incoming Soul continues to make his presence felt.

The mother At this time the woman usually feels at her best. Both she and her baby are growing well and healthily.

Landmark At some time during this trimester the woman will feel her baby moving.

The hormones By the mid-trimester the levels of HCG have decreased and the mother feels better. Oestrogen and Progesterone increase in quantity with the main production in the placenta. The placenta produces many hormones to support the pregnancy; they include Human Chorionic Somatomammotropin (HCS), Human Placental Lactogen (HPL) and Relaxin.

Reflexology The greatest work of the reflexologist is done at this time - to support the natural development of a mother-to-be and a new life.
Give full reflexology sessions and reflexology therapy for any minor ailments if appropriate.

THE THIRD TRIMESTER OF PREGNANCY

The third trimester is the last three months of pregnancy or from week 28 until birthing.

The Incoming Soul The baby is considered viable from 24 weeks gestation. He has everything he needs - all he has to do is grow both in size and maturity.

The mother The mother also grows! During the last few weeks of pregnancy the woman can feel great discomfort and long for it all to be over.

The hormones During the third trimester the hormones of pregnancy keep increasing. At the end of the pregnancy Progesterone levels diminish and the hormones of birthing take effect.

Reflexology Ideally reflexology sessions once a week help the woman keep up with the hormonal changes and help prepare her for birthing.
It is better to give shorter more frequent sessions.
Include more relaxation techniques, balancing and harmonising grips, gentle stretches especially the pelvic stretches, endocrine balance and reflexology lymphatic technique.

Caution

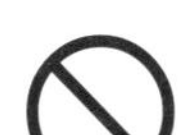

When positioning the woman for a session, ensure that she is NOT lying flat. If she lies flat the weight of her baby may press on her inferior vena cava and lower her blood pressure.

Cautions

There seems to be a general feeling of anxiety about working with pregnant clients especially in early pregnancy.

Learning reflexology — It is wise that whilst learning reflexology students are recommended to NOT work with pregnant clients during the first trimester.

Rationale — There is so much to learn during reflexology training and extra knowledge is needed for working with pregnant clients.

This next section will deal with some worries and fears to clarify for the reflexologist which ones are genuine and which can be explained.

CATEGORIES FOR CAUTION

There are two main categories with reasons to omit reflexology therapy during pregnancy.

A) If the practitioner does not want to do it.

B) If the client does not want it done.

All the reasons fall into these two categories.

A) SOME REASONS WHY THE PRACTITIONER MAY NOT WANT TO "DO" REFLEXOLOGY

- Fear that it may cause miscarriage.
- Fear that it may damage the foetus.
- Fear of litigation.
- It is against the obstetric caregiver's orders.
- A feeling of inexperience.
- She/he has been taught not to work with clients during the first trimester of pregnancy.
- An unexplained sense of not-to-do-it-ness a "felt sense".

B) SOME REASONS WHY THE PREGNANT CLIENT MAY NOT WANT TO HAVE REFLEXOLOGY

- She has heard that it is:
  - painful
  - can cause miscarriage
  - that there are terrible reactions.
- People in her life like her husband, father, doctor, friends either poo-poo the idea or are unsupportive or hostile.
- She does not like her feet being touched.
- It is too expensive.

CONSIDERATION OF REASONS FOR CAUTION

Some reasons why the practitioner may not want to "do" reflexology.

FEAR THAT IT MAY CAUSE MISCARRIAGE

Viable foetus

If there is a viable foetus it is extremely difficult to dislodge it.
Mother Nature is irrepressible in her campaign to aid reproduction; it is of the greatest importance that the species continues.

Miscarriage is a natural occurrence

About 98% of all early miscarriages are caused by chromosomal abnormalities in the foetus.

Reflexology

If there is a risk of foetal loss due to other causes, such as habitual miscarriage, when the client has reflexology her being is more balanced and so there is a good possibility that she will be able to maintain her pregnancy.

FEAR THAT IT MAY DAMAGE THE FOETUS

Known things that damage the foetus

- Drugs
- Alcohol
- Smoking
- Diet (lack of folic acid)
- Genetic flaw

Reflexology

Reflexology does not enter that list.

FEAR OF LITIGATION

Distressed clients

Some clients may experience a problem during their pregnancy and attribute it to the reflexologist.
There will always be distressed people.

Reflexologist

Always work with your own truth, love, caring, skills and knowledge.

Protect your back, observe the contraindications and take the necessary precautions.

Always keep records that can stand up to legal examination. That is, write them up immediately after the reflexology session, date and sign them and retain them for 21 years.

IT IS AGAINST THE OBSTETRIC CARER'S ORDERS

The obstetric caregiver

The obstetric caregiver is obliged to client confidentially and must not discuss his/her client. There may be occasions when there are reasons to withhold complementary care - the reflexologist is advised to respect the obstetric caregiver's wishes.

Assumption of hostility

It is often assumed that the medical profession is hostile to complementary therapies. An occasional one may be hostile, however most medical practitioners are open to things that are beneficial to their patients.

Reflexologist

It is important that the obstetric team is given information of the benefits of reflexology. Good communication can often solve the problem of apparent hostility.
Communication can also help the unsupportive or hostile people in the client's life.

A FEELING OF INEXPERIENCE

Solve this problem

The best way to solve this problem is to get some experience.

Reflexologist

Trust the therapy to be beneficial, observe the contraindications and enjoy the experience of working with pregnant feet.

AN UNEXPLAINED SENSE OF "NOT-TO-DO-IT-NESS" AN "UNCLEAR FELT SENSE"

Top of the list

This reason for not working with clients in the first trimester is most important and needs to be at the **top** of the list.

Reflexologist

Always listen to your seventh sense. You may never know the reason - just trust your intuition.

With the above information, consider how best to respond to the client's reasons for NOT wanting reflexology during pregnancy:

- She has heard that it is:
    - painful
    - can cause miscarriage
    - that there are terrible reactions.
- People in her life such as her husband, father, doctor, friends either poo-poo the idea and are unsupportive or hostile.
- She does not like her feet being touched.
- It is too expensive.

CONTRAINDICATIONS

There are some occasions when reflexology is contraindicated:

- Acupressure points.
- Deep Vein Thrombosis.

ACUPRESSURE POINTS

There are three acupressure points that are traditionally forbidden to use during pregnancy as they may cause an interruption of pregnancy. They are located within the foot reflexology area.

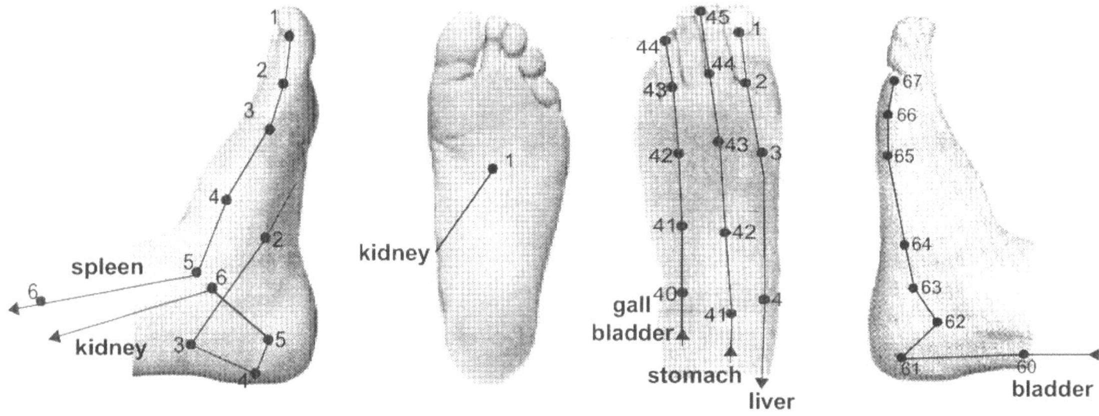

Spleen 6

This is one of the most important acupuncture points for the reproductive system.

Spleen 6:

- Harmonises Blood and energy flows of the reproductive system. (David Tai)
- Moves Blood too strongly. (Yana Stanjyo)
- Frees Blood stasis in the uterus. If stimulated in the first three months of pregnancy will cause a spontaneous abortion of the foetus. (Meridian Therapy Ryodoraku)
- Produces a downward movement of Qi causing expulsion of the uterine contents. (Acupuncture in Midwifery, Sharon Yelland)

Bladder 60

Expedites labour. (John Allan p12)

Bladder 67

Expedites labour. (John Allan p12)

Caution

Hand reflexology: Reflexologists doing hand reflexology must check for any acupressure points in the hands that may need to be avoided during pregnancy.

DEEP VEIN THROMBOSIS (DVT)

DVT is a blood clot that forms inside a vein. It may partially or completely block the blood flow. There is a risk that fragments may detach and travel to another part of the body causing an embolus e.g. pulmonary embolus. The thrombosis can occur in any deep vein. The vein most often affected is the deep vein in the calf - the deep saphenous.

Note

Pregnant women are more prone to have DVT than are any other groups of people.

Physiology

During pregnancy the high levels of oestrogens are associated with DVT. The natural physiology when good blood clotting is necessary to prepare the body for birthing can aggravate DVT.
Increasing weight impedes the venous return from the legs.

Contraindication

STOP

As reflexology increases the vitality of the vascular system there is a possibility that the thrombosis may move with dire consequences.

Therefore DO NOT "do" reflexology with clients who have DVT.

Signs & symptoms

Locally:

- Pain
- Swelling
- Heat
- Redness

Sometimes the client may complain of cramp or there may be no sign at all.

Test for DVT

Dorsiflex the foot. If a DVT is present there is excruciating pain - a positive Homan's sign.

Action

DO NOT REPEAT THE TEST

DO NOT MOVE THE CLIENT

SEEK MEDICAL ASSISTANCE IMMEDIATELY

Reflexology Techniques

ADAPTING REFLEXOLOGY TECHNIQUES FOR PREGNANCY

BIMANUAL "SOLAR PLEXUS" HOLD

This is a hold that accesses one of the most important points on the foot. In reflexology it reflects the centre of the base of the lungs and part of the diaphragm.

Point of interest

In Traditional Chinese Medicine (TCM) the same area is the start of the Kidney meridian (K1). This is the place where the life creative force enters the body. It is especially useful during pregnancy as the mother's life force (chi) is dedicated to creating the pre-natal chi of the Incoming Soul.

Acupressure point K1 is used for extreme fear, severe anxiety and shock.

Method

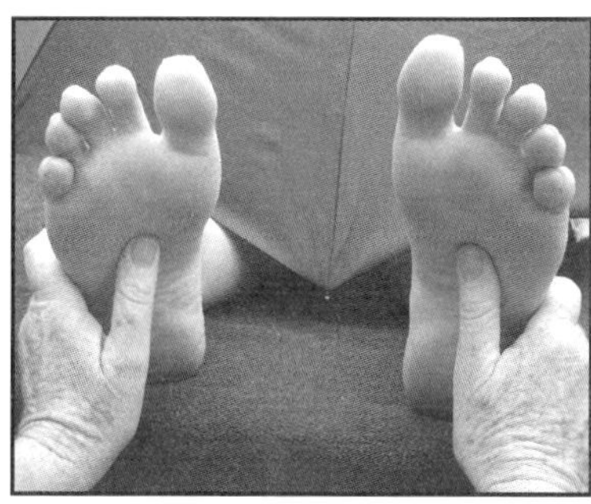

Place both thumbs simultaneously on the "solar plexus" reflex zones, rest the fingers where they naturally fall and hold this position until the client is calmer. This may take one to ten minutes.

Variations

- Slightly rotate the thumbs together with right thumb moving anti-clockwise and left thumb moving clockwise to "unwind" the energy.
- Slightly rotate the thumbs together with right thumb moving clockwise and left thumb moving anti-clockwise to "wind-up" the energy.
- Whilst holding "solar plexus" reflex zone, gently rock from side to side the entirety of both feet.
- Send a vibration through the thumbs.
- Gently pump.
- Use your own "solar plexus" hand reflex zone anywhere over the client's foot as a healing hold.

Uses

- Calming, settling, grounding.
- Re-energising.
- Extreme fear, severe anxiety and shock.
- Panic attacks.
- To reinforce the mother's creative life force.

SPINAL TWIST

This movement mimics the yoga spinal twist.

Method

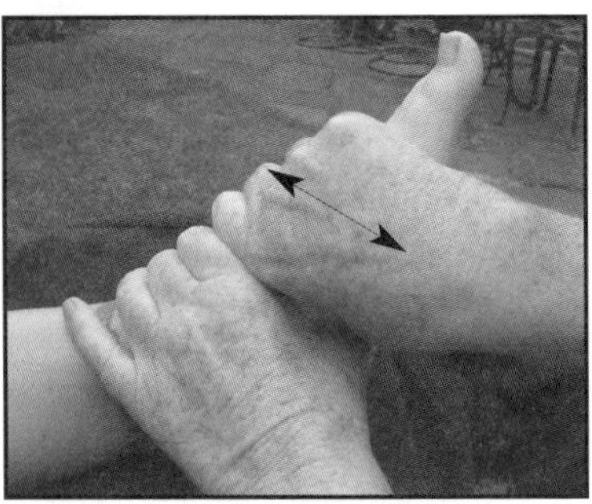

With palms facing down, put both hands together with the index fingers side by side and the thumbs pointing down. Keep the hands together and take hold of a foot as near to the ankle as possible. The webbing between the thumb and index finger is around the instep. The hand nearest the ankle holds the foot firmly; the hand nearest the toes twists the foot away then back and returns it to its original position. Both hands together shuffle a tiny bit towards the toes. Repeat the twist and shuffle until the whole spine reflex zone has been worked. Repeat on the other foot.

Pregnancy adaptation

During the second and third trimesters it may be uncomfortable for the client to be grasped by her abdominal reflex zone.
This movement is too good for her to miss out on.
To adapt it to pregnancy, hold the same way but with the thumbs resting lightly.
To get the twist push the lateral side of the foot down with the ends of the fingers and to return use the webbing between thumbs and index fingers.

Uses

- Enhance the vitality of the back.
- Tired back.
- Aching back and belly muscles.

SPINAL RUB

This movement mimics the experience of having your back rubbed dry with a fresh hot towel.

Method

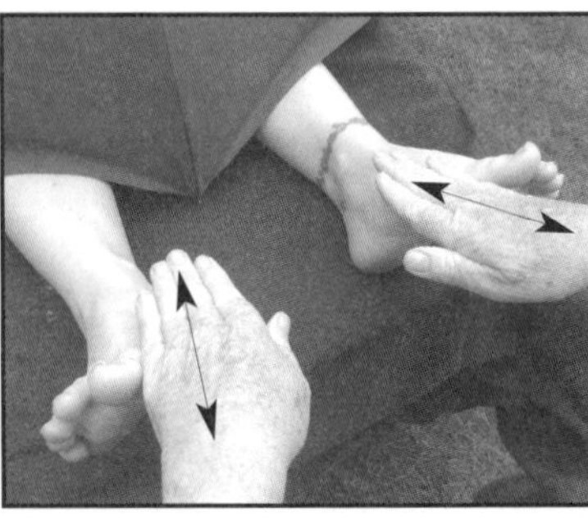

With palms facing down angle the hands at 45° with fingers down. Place the sides of little fingers against the cervical vertebrae reflex zones. Use a sawing movement and progressively move down the medial side of the foot. **At the same time** progressively use more of the hands and arms, i.e. the side of the small finger for the cervical vertebrae reflex zones, the side of the hands for the thoracic vertebrae reflex zones, the small finger, the side of the hands and the side of the forearm for the lumbar vertebrae reflex zones and from the small finger to the elbow for the inner pelvic reflex zones.

Uses

- Pleasure.
- Increase the vitality for a tired back.
- Ease backache.

FISH / RIPPLE

Created by Susanne Enzer especially to use during birthing to prevent the toes pulling back.

Method

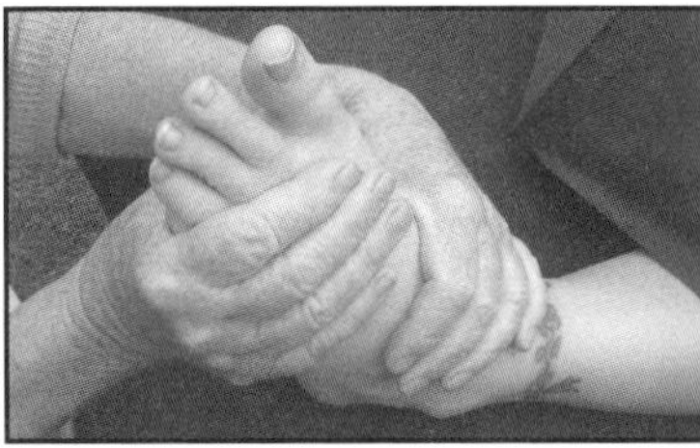

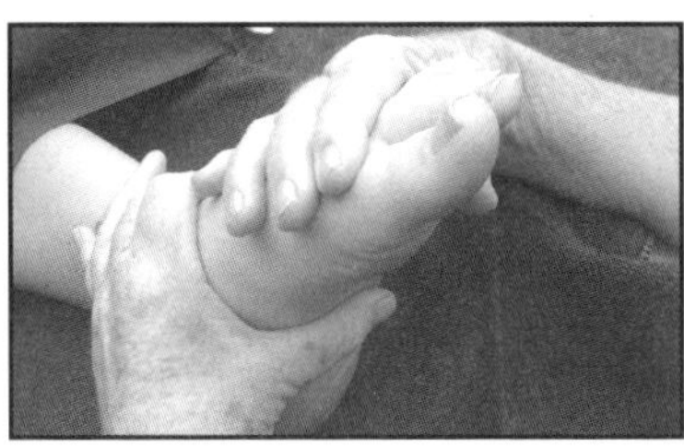

With the left hand use a firm, steadying grip on the left foot. Using the right hand hold the foot with the thumb across the ball of the foot and the fingers across the back of the foot, the webbing of the thumb and index finger around the joint of the little toe and the foot. Create a ripple across the shoulder girdle reflex zone. To do this the two extremes of the movement are: twist the shoulder reflex zone by pushing away with the thumb and pulling towards you with the webbing and another twist press towards you with the fingers and push away with the webbing. Soften the movement between the two extremes.

Variations

Use the same movement to include the toes.
Bimanually, use one hand on each foot.

Uses

- To ease shoulder tension.
- First stage of labour.

LUNG PRESS

This technique imitates the movement of respiration.

Method

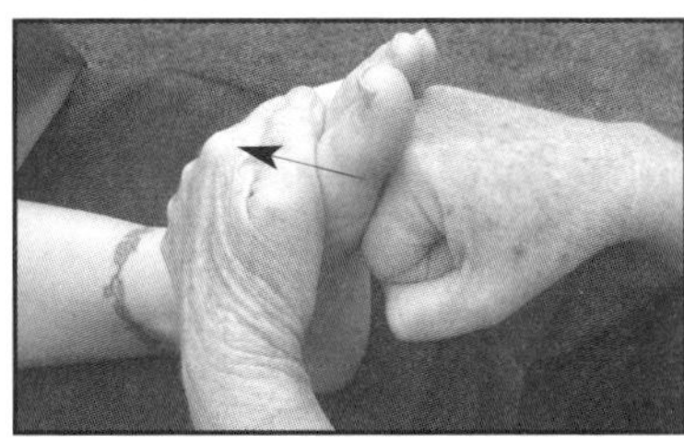

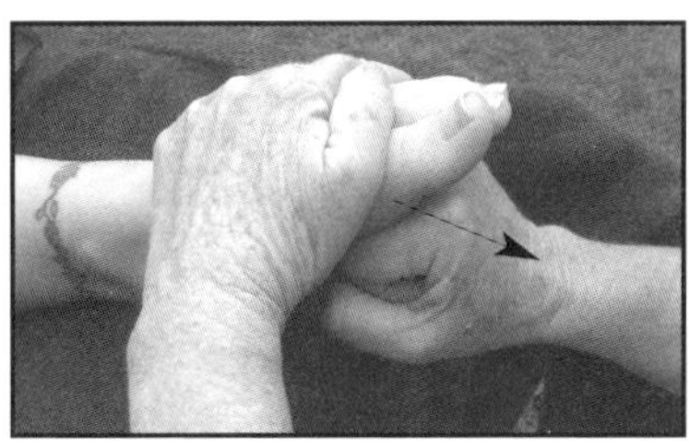

With right hand make a fist. Place the fingers part of the fist flat on the ball of the foot, with the knuckles in line with the shoulder girdle reflex zone. Place the left hand across the back of the foot, leaving the toes exposed. With the fist push the foot towards the client, and then with the left hand squeeze the sides of the foot at the same time pull it back down. Create rhythmical movements.

The push movement mimics inspiration, the pull movement mimics expiration.

Because this technique mimics the movements of respiration it can be used to influence respiration of the client.

Variations

Do the push / pull movement in time with the client's breathing to maintain steady respirations.
Do the push / pull movement at a normal respiration rate to obtain a steady respiration rate.

Uses

- Emotional upsets.
- Hyperventilation or panic attacks.
- First stage of labour.

PELVIC STRETCH

This movement mimics the position of the hips and pelvis when squatting.

Method

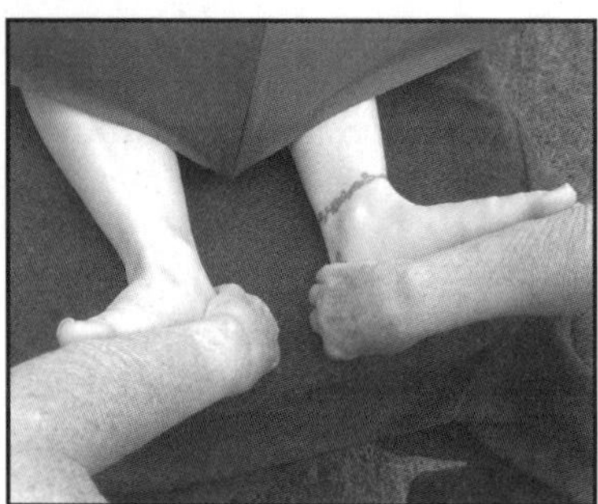

Tuck the fingers of both hands under both heels. Rest forearms on the medial side of the plantar aspect of the feet. Lean onto the feet gently pushing them back and out.

Uses

- Preparation for birthing.
- Preconceptual care.
- Dysmenorrhoea.
- During birthing if the client cannot squat.
- After a traumatic vaginal delivery.

ANKLE BOOGIE also known as ANKLE LOOSENER

During pregnancy use this technique in moderation and do it slowly and gently.

Uses

To maintain the flexibility of the pelvis.

Precaution

This technique is too strong for the first trimester of pregnancy if done vigorously.

ANKLE ROTATIONS

Use this technique frequently.

Uses

- To maintain the flexibility of the pelvis.
- To assess the flexibility of the pelvis.
- This is a useful technique for easing dysmenorrhoea and for preconceptual relaxation.

THUMB AND FINGER WALKING TECHNIQUES

Use positive but gentle movements.

Precaution

Do NOT use vigorous or deeply probing movements especially on the internal pelvic reflex zones and some acupressure points.

SPECIAL TECHNIQUES

URINARY SYSTEM "FLUSH"

During pregnancy it is important to treat the kidneys very gently. This technique uses a gently stroking movement that follows the direction of urine flow - from kidneys, through ureters, bladder and urethra.

Method

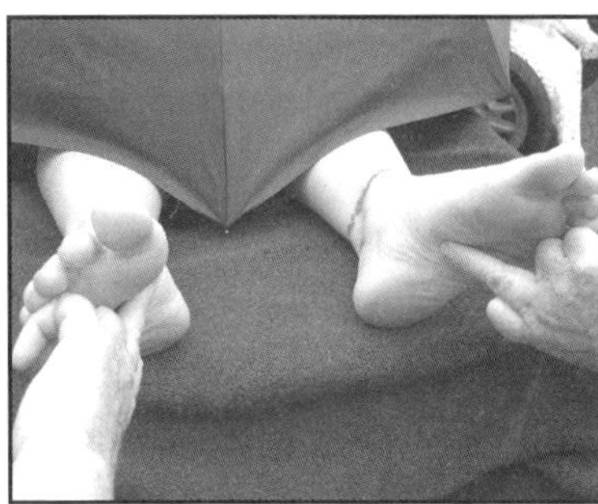

Use middle fingers. Begin by placing the pads of both fingers on both kidney reflex zones. Stroke gently but firmly along the length of the urinary system reflex zones. The same movement may be done using thumbs instead of third fingers.

Uses

- Use with every reflexology session to maintain health.
- In conjunction with the reflexology lymphatic technique.
- For hypertensive clients.
- Clients with micturition problems.

REFLEXOLOGY RELATED TECHNIQUES

The following techniques do not form part of this learning, however they may be used safely and effectively with pregnant clients.

Linking Technique

This is a very gentle method of using subtle energies. Prue Hughes, Principal of the School of Precision Reflexology in Devon, England created this technique. Prue says, *"Linking is an effective technique for enhancing reflexology treatments. It is complementary to any method already practiced, is safe to use and gives power and precision to the treatment. It is a safe method as we are linking into the client's own healing energies."*.

Brazilian Balance

This is a technique that has been described by Rex Myers and Peter Eedy. It seems to use the subtle energies in the toes to align the longitudinal zones of the body.

Metamorphic Technique

Gaston Saint Pierre developed this technique from a system of change or Metamorphosis that was created by an Australian reflexologist, Robert St John. Part of the technique includes the "Pre-natal Pattern" where the spine reflex zones record the events of the time of gestation.

Recommended reading

The Metamorphic Technique, by Gaston Saint Pierre.

SOME LESSER KNOWN REFLEX ZONES

"SENSE OF SELF"

The second toes hold the awareness of the "Sense of Self". Valerie Barton, an Australian reflexologist with her insight and intuition originated this reflex zone. She says that "the "Sense of Self" is a sense that "I" am part of the Greater Scheme of Things, a sense of Spirit within". The author has an understanding that in Traditional Chinese Medicine (TCM) there is a concept that the Spirit resides in the Heart. The second toe is the loving toe and has connection with the chest area, which includes the heart.

Uses — To give inner strength to the client when she feels that she has lost herself in childbearing, birthing and motherhood.

"BALANCE ORGAN"

The "Balance Organ" is located on both feet, on the dorsal aspect at the distal end in the groove between metatarsals four and five. Father Joseph Euguster describes the "Balance Organ" in the book Rwo Shur Health Method as being "applicable to dizziness, vertigo, car- and sea-sickness and balance problems" (p98). In TCM it is the acupressure point Gall Bladder 42.

Uses — This point is particularly helpful when a client is emotionally "out of balance". The "Balance organ" may be used in conjunction with other reflex zones and may be linked to the heart, head, "solar plexus" or pelvic reflex zones.

"COPING POINT"

The "Coping Point" is located on both feet on the dorsal aspect of the webbing between the second and third toes. Devaki Berkson in her book 'The Foot Book" identifies the "Coping Point" (p98). In TCM it is the acupressure point Stomach 44.

Uses — This point is useful when the client's coping ability needs a boost. the "Coping Point" may be used in conjunction with other reflex zones and may be linked to the heart, head, "solar plexus" or pelvic reflex zones.

Reflexology Pregnancy Care

Author's opinion

In the opinion of the author reflexology is second to none for pregnancy care!

Natural therapy

Reflexology as a natural therapy complements the natural event of childbearing.

Holistic modality

It is an holistic modality that encompasses body, mind and spirit.

Reflexologists' knowledge

Reflexologists who have been working in this field know that reflexology increases health and well being and gives an excellent environment for both mother and the Incoming Soul. It reduces stress and anxiety, which can cause problems.

Research project

A research project undertaken by Dr Gowrie Motha in London *"discovered that the effects of reflexology (during the antenatal period) on labour outcomes were outstanding".* (See page 178 for list of articles & research)

Fantastic experience

Pregnancy, especially the first one, is a fantastic experience. Astounding changes happen to women during pregnancy. Every body system is involved - so are the emotions and feelings.

Pregnant women adapt

Usually pregnant women adapt well to the changes in body and mind and make the most of the experience.

Minor ailments

Some women experience discomfort and minor ailments, which respond well to reflexology therapy.

Major problems

Occasionally minor ailments develop into complications, disorders and major obstetric problems that must have expert medical attention.

Reflexologist

Maternity reflexology is wonderful work.
Enjoy the experience.

Caution

ALL problems during pregnancy MUST have expert medical attention.

GENERAL WELLBEING

Reflexology sessions

In an ideal situation a reflexology session each week throughout pregnancy is the best way to maintain balance and harmony during the rapidly changing condition of pregnancy. Unfortunately this is neither possible nor practical.

Shorter sessions

Consider working shorter sessions. Little and often is a good scheme.

Client comfort

For client comfort use a reclining chair rather than a massage couch. The client may be too cumbersome to climb onto a couch and she will need to use the toilet frequently.

Precaution

Remember to never let her lie flat on her back. (Supine Hypotension).

Always include

In each session always include:

- Endocrine system balance.
- Reflexology lymphatic technique.
- "Solar plexus" hold.
- Reflexology therapy for disordered zones (if appropriate).

Body Systems

The following information is arranged in body systems.

Each system includes

- Diagram of the anatomical placement and reflex zones.
- Simple pregnancy physiology.
- Some metaphysical aspects.
- General reflexology to maintain the vitality of the system.

Some problems

- A definition of the problem.
- Simple physiology of how the problem may have occurred.
- Cautions to be aware of when the minor ailment becomes a major problem.
- Suggested reflexology to **include in the session**.

Reflex zones

When part of the anatomy is named in the reflexology therapy tables please assume that it is the foot reflex zone unless otherwise stated.

Recommended resource

Maternity Reflexology Pregnancy Care Reference Cards, by Susanne Enzer, Soul to Sole Reflexology.

SKELETAL SYSTEM

ANATOMICAL PLACEMENT AND REFLEX ZONES

RIGHT PLANTAR ASPECT | FRONT OF SKELETON | LEFT PLANTAR ASPECT

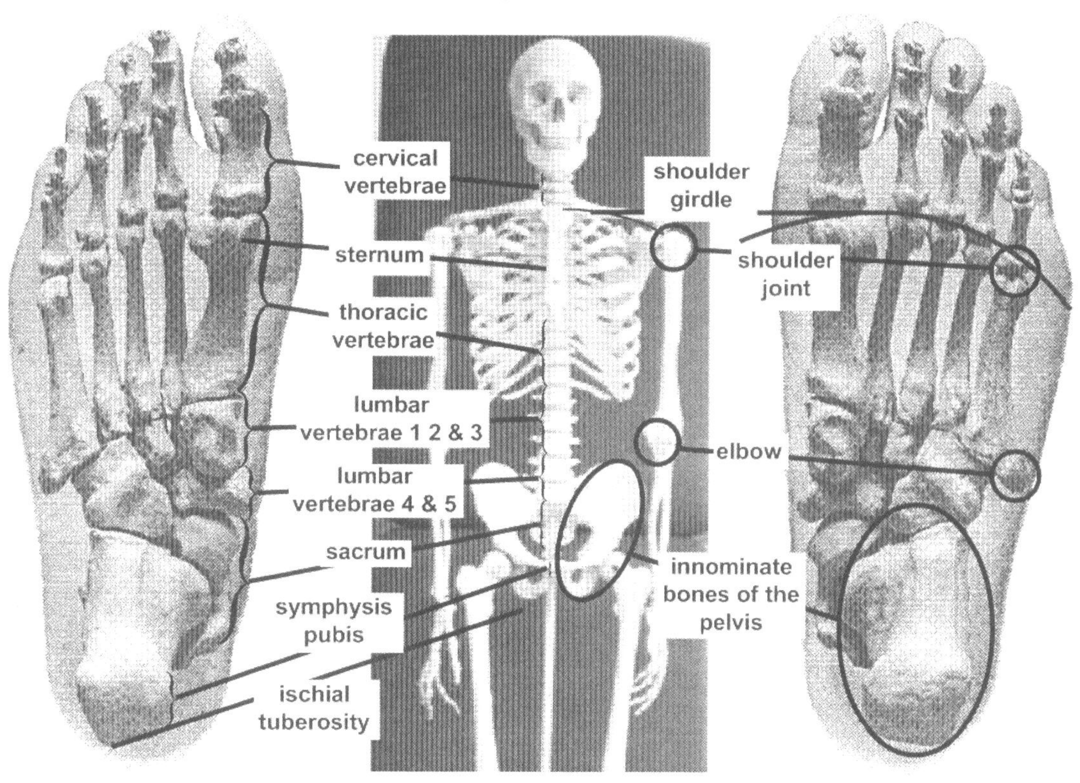

Physiology

The effects of increasing weight, altered stance, change of pelvic tilt and the pregnancy hormones especially relaxin, put a great strain on the musculo-skeletal system.

Metaphysical aspects

The skeleton not only provides a solid foundation and a framework for the body but also for life.
The spine holds the support in life.
Shoulders carry loads.
Sternum (breast bone) holds strength and invincibility.
Hips hold stability in movement.
Atlas, sacrum and talus are weight bearers.

Reflexology

Maintain the vitality of the system.
Spine relaxing and stretching techniques.

Old Wive's Tale

It is an old wives tale that "women loose a tooth for each pregnancy". The truth behind this tale is that the baby makes a great demand on calcium to grow his bones and if the mother is not having adequate nutrition he will acquire his calcium from her bones or teeth.

BACKACHE

Backache is discomfort or pain in the back.

Physiology	The back muscles work hard to compensate for the increasing weight of the baby. As the baby grows the woman leans back to counterbalance the weight and realign her centre of gravity. The pregnancy hormone relaxin causes the ligaments in the back to soften.
Metaphysical aspects	The spine holds the support in life. Upper back holds emotional support for loving and nurturing. Middle back holds deep emotional support for subconscious events. Lower back holds physical support. Backache may be related to lack of support in those areas.
Minor ailment	Although backache is unpleasant it is considered to be one of the pregnancy aches and pains.
MAJOR PROBLEM	Backache becomes a major problem when it is extremely painful and incapacitating.
Reflexology	
Spine	Spine stretches - to ease the discomfort. Pregnancy adapted spinal twist - to keep the joints supple. Massage type movements - to re-establish support.
Head & neck	Stretch and rotate - to lengthen the spine.
Diaphragm	Diaphragm work - to ease emotional stress.
Extra advice	Advise the client to rest for short periods whenever possible as well as using good lifting techniques at all times. Recommend that she practice her back, abdomen and pelvic floor exercises regularly.

RIB PAIN

Rib pain is pain in the lower border of the ribs.

Physiology	The normal change in the rib cage due to pregnancy is an increase in the subcostal angle. Towards the end of pregnancy, as the baby grows and the uterus enlarges it pushes up under the ribs. The softening affect of the hormone relaxin and the stretching of the abdominal muscles attached to the ribs cause the ribs to separate and create a constant dull pain. The condition is aggravated if the baby is in a breech position.
Minor ailment	Rib pain is very uncomfortable but not a major problem. The problem will be relieved when the baby's head engages in the pelvis and makes more space under the ribs. This condition is unlikely to become a major problem; however recommend that the client inform her obstetric caregiver to ensure that the chest pain is in fact rib pain.
Extra advice	Consult a kinesiologist, as there are areas along the lower ribs called "alarm points" that may be disordered.
Reflexology	
Shoulder girdle	Relaxation techniques - to ease the tension.
Spine	Spine stretches - to give a little more abdominal space. Pregnancy adapted spinal twist - to increase mobility.
Lungs	Lung press - to re-establish balanced respirations.
Diaphragm	Diaphragm work - to ease emotional stress.
Extra advice	Remind the client to maintain good posture and laugh as much as possible!

SYMPHYSIS PUBIS PAIN

Symphysis pubis pain is also known as separated symphysis or diastasis of symphysis pubis or pathological laxity of the symphysis pubis. It is a disabling disorder with pain in the pubic area that is severe when walking.

Physiology

The effect of the hormone relaxin increases the laxity of the pubic joint, which may cause separation of the pubic bones.

Precaution
Possible major problem

A client with any severe pain especially in the reproductive system must be advised to see her obstetric caregiver.

Once a diagnosis of separated symphysis has been made reflexology treatments may be commenced.

Reflexology First Aid

Symphysis pubis

For three consecutive days do the Trigger Point Release reflexology technique on the reflex zones of the symphysis pubis for two minutes each. This has been found to be very effective in reducing / relieving pain (see page 159).

"Solar plexus"

Bi-manual "solar plexus" hold - to relieve anxiety.

Caution

The Trigger Point Release technique is not suitable for most reflex zones during pregnancy. This is one exception. Ensure absolute accuracy of the location of the reflex zones.

REPRODUCTIVE SYSTEM

ANATOMICAL PLACEMENT & REFLEX ZONES

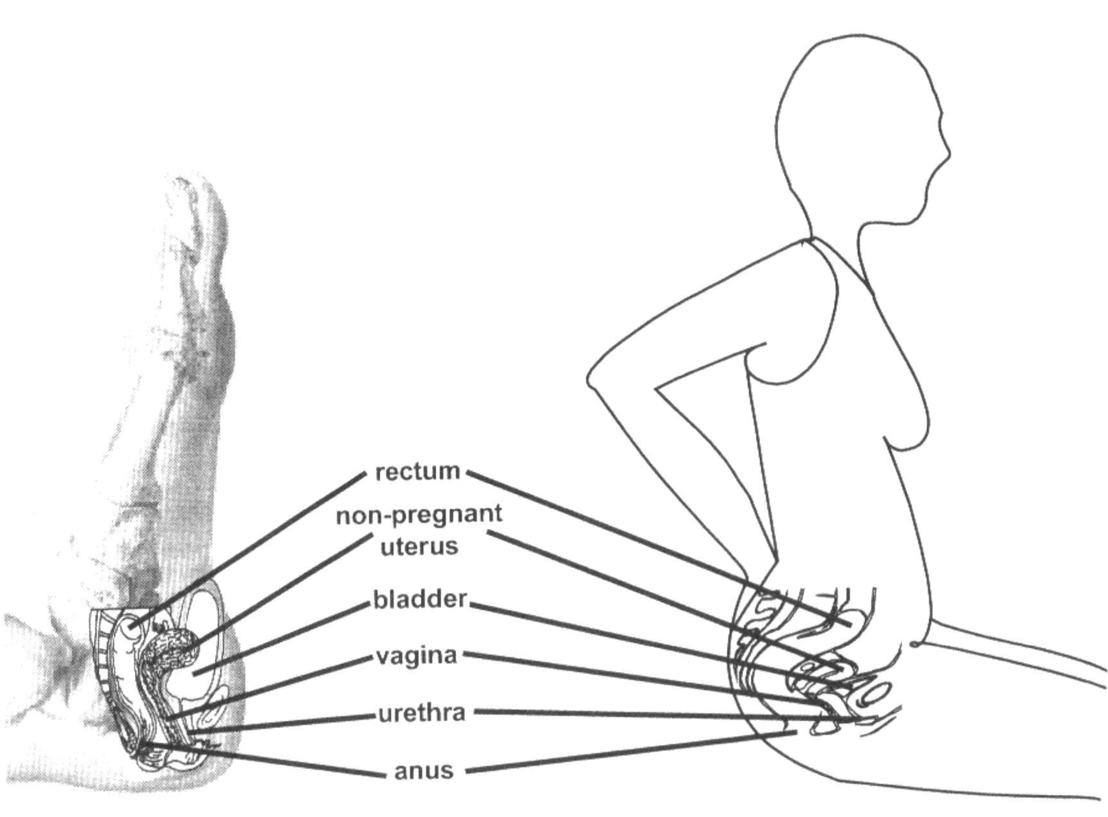

Physiology

The uterus is an amazing organ. At the start of pregnancy it is about the size of a closed fist. At the end of pregnancy the uterus has increased 2,200% in size. To enable this enormous change it lays down more muscle and increases the blood flow.

Metaphysical aspects

The effect of the mind and emotions are held in the soft tissue of the body.

The uterus represents the home of creativity. It is related to space and boundaries; during pregnancy it provides a warm supportive environment and at the same time has the ability to expand with changing demands made of it.

Reflexology

Give gentle care acknowledging the greatness of these organs.

MISCARRIAGE

Miscarriage or spontaneous abortion of the pregnancy is the passing of the foetus and all or part of the placenta during the first twenty weeks of pregnancy. There are many causes for miscarriage.

THREATENED MISCARRIAGE	Threatened miscarriage is vaginal bleeding which is often painless.
INEVITABLE MISCARRIAGE	Inevitable miscarriage is when the vaginal bleeding continues accompanied by discomfort / pain. The cervix opens and it is inevitable that the foetus will be passed.
INCOMPLETE MISCARRIAGE	Incomplete miscarriage is when the foetus is passed but part or all of the placenta remains. Bleeding continues until the placenta is removed.
MISSED ABORTION	Missed abortion is when the foetus dies but the woman does not miscarry.
HABITUAL or RECURRENT MISCARRIAGE	This term applies to women who have had three previous miscarriages.
PRE-TERM LABOUR	After twenty weeks gestation if the woman goes into labour it is not considered to be a miscarriage but pre-term labour.

Caution — **All of the above conditions require medical attention.**

Many reflexologists prefer to not work with clients in these categories. However, knowing that nothing will change the outcome, reflexologists can support their client who will be experiencing a very unpleasant and frightening time.

Note — By "doing" reflexology with a client who has recurrent miscarriages, it will balance the being so she has a better chance of maintaining her pregnancy.

EARLY MISCARRIAGE
In very early pregnancy many miscarriages occur without the woman being aware that she has become pregnant. She may think that her period was "a bit late" and "a bit heavy" and pay no further attention to it.

Reflexology	General reflexology.

FIRST TRIMESTER MISCARRIAGE
A first trimester miscarriage is always an emotional time for the woman even with an unplanned or unwanted pregnancy. The loss of a wanted or long awaited precious pregnancy is devastating

Reflexology	General reflexology, especially an endocrine balance and the reflexology lymphatic technique. Listening skills.

SECOND TRIMESTER MISCARRIAGE
A late miscarriage is a truly grievous event.

Reflexology	General reflexology, especially an endocrine balance and the reflexology lymphatic technique. Listening skills, great care, concern and loving kindness.

Note — Be prepared to cry.

AFTER MISCARRIAGE OR TERMINATION OF PREGNANCY

Although this is not pregnancy care it is included here for reflexologists who have worked with a client during the time before their miscarriage or termination of pregnancy and want to keep on caring for their client.

Losing a baby	Losing a baby is always an emotional time. A period of grieving is to be expected when feelings of denial, anger / and or guilt are expressed.
Termination of pregnancy (TOP)	TOP is not usually used as a form of contraception. It is a very difficult decision to be made. There is often concealment and guilt. Sometimes the client herself does not make the decision and she is obliged to comply with another person's decision. Sometimes the client knows that her decision to terminate her pregnancy was the wrong choice. The ongoing effects of TOP can disrupt a woman's life for many years. For instance she may have difficulty conceiving when she wants to. If she has concealed it the guilt may stay with her till her dying day.
Note	There is no time limit for the care of a client who has lost a baby; it may be immediate or many years later. When taking a client history it is worth asking about TOP; you may be the only person who has done so.
Extra care	If it has not been done already suggest a closing ritual that includes a name for the baby and a meaningful farewell.

Reflexology	
Endocrine system	Endocrine balance - to help restore the non-pregnant hormonal balance.
Non-pregnant uterus, indirect ovary and "solar plexus"	Linking technique - to reconnect the energy.
Hypothalamus and "sense of self"	Linking technique - to help her find herself again.
"Solar plexus"	Hold - to calm, centre and restore the creative life force.
Lower abdomen and internal pelvis	Healing hold - to help prevent feelings of guilt settling.
Lymphatic system	Lymphatic technique - to help cleanse the body.

GROIN PAIN / LIGAMENT PAIN

Groin pain / ligament pain is a sharp pain that feels like a "stitch". It may occur on both sides of the body, but more frequently it occurs on the right side.

Physiology	The baby grows at his own rate. The uterus grows to accommodate the baby. The ligaments (round ligaments) do not always stretch at the same time causing the pain.
Minor ailment	This condition is a discomfort and can be frightening for the client, but in itself is not dangerous. The sharp pain episodes usually pass in a few days.
Problem	A client with any severe pain especially in the reproductive system must be advised to see her obstetric caregiver.

Reflexology	
Abdomen	Relaxation techniques - to relax and allow the ligament to stretch.
Spine	Relaxation techniques - to lessen tension and increase mobility.
"Solar plexus"	Hold - to relieve anxiety.
Note	Sometimes the reflexion of the tight ligament can be palpated on the foot. It feels like a thin piece of string running diagonally from about longitudinal zone 5 at the waistline to longitudinal zone 1 on the groin line. Usually on the right foot. Using both thumbs: do a movement like stretching an elastic band on the reflection of the tight ligament.

BRAXTON HICKS CONTRACTIONS

Braxton Hicks contractions are uterine contractions that are irregular and increase in frequency and intensity as pregnancy advances. They are part of the normal progress of pregnancy.

Physiology

The uterus responds to the placental hormones by contracting and relaxing.

Minor ailment

Most women are delighted to feel these contractions. Occasionally a client may perceive them to be a minor ailment.

PRE-TERM LABOUR

Pre-term labour is labour that begins before the end of the thirty-seventh week of pregnancy. Braxton Hicks contractions may become regular and increase in intensity and turn into pre-term labour contractions.

Physiology

In most cases no obvious reason can be found for pre-term labour, but the commonest causes are pre-eclampsia, ante-partum haemorrhage and multiple pregnancy.

MAJOR PROBLEM

The baby

Pre-term babies, (those born before 36 weeks gestation) are immature and can have great problems with their lungs and bowels. They have poor or absent sucking reflex and many other problems. These little souls need very specialised care and can generally do very well.

The mother

Must have immediate obstetric care.

Caution

Before commencing reflexology, this client MUST be in a place where should she birth her baby there is access to specialised baby care.

Reflexology

Entire body

All relaxation techniques with extreme gentleness - to relax the entire being.

"Solar plexus"

Hold - to calm extreme fear, anxiety and terror.

Note

These deceptively simple techniques can be most effective.

VAGINAL BLEEDING

Caution

DURING PREGNANCY THERE SHOULD BE NO VAGINAL BLEEDING

IMPLANTATION BLEEDING

Implantation bleeding occurs when the fertilised ovum embeds itself in the lining of the uterus.
It may be mistaken for a light menstrual period.
The problem associated with this is that there may be a miscalculation of the expected date of delivery (EDD).
It is not dangerous to the pregnancy.

SPOTTING

Spotting is a commonly used term for when a client has small vaginal bleeds throughout her pregnancy. Once the obstetric caregiver has assessed the client and the bleeding found to be benign, it is acceptable to "do" reflexology.

MISCARRIAGE

Vaginal bleeding and pain occur prior to miscarriage. These clients need obstetric / gynaecological care. (See miscarriage, page 64).

ANTEPARTUM HAEMORRHAGE

Antepartum haemorrhage is potentially life threatening to both mother and baby.

MAJOR OBSTETRIC PROBLEM

These clients need immediate obstetric care.

Caution

Except for the client who has implantation bleeding the reflexologist would be well advised to have the obstetric caregiver's written permission to "do" reflexology.

Reflexology First Aid
"Solar plexus"

Hold - to calm extreme anxiety, fear and panic.

ALIMENTARY SYSTEM

ANATOMICAL PLACEMENT AND REFLEX ZONES

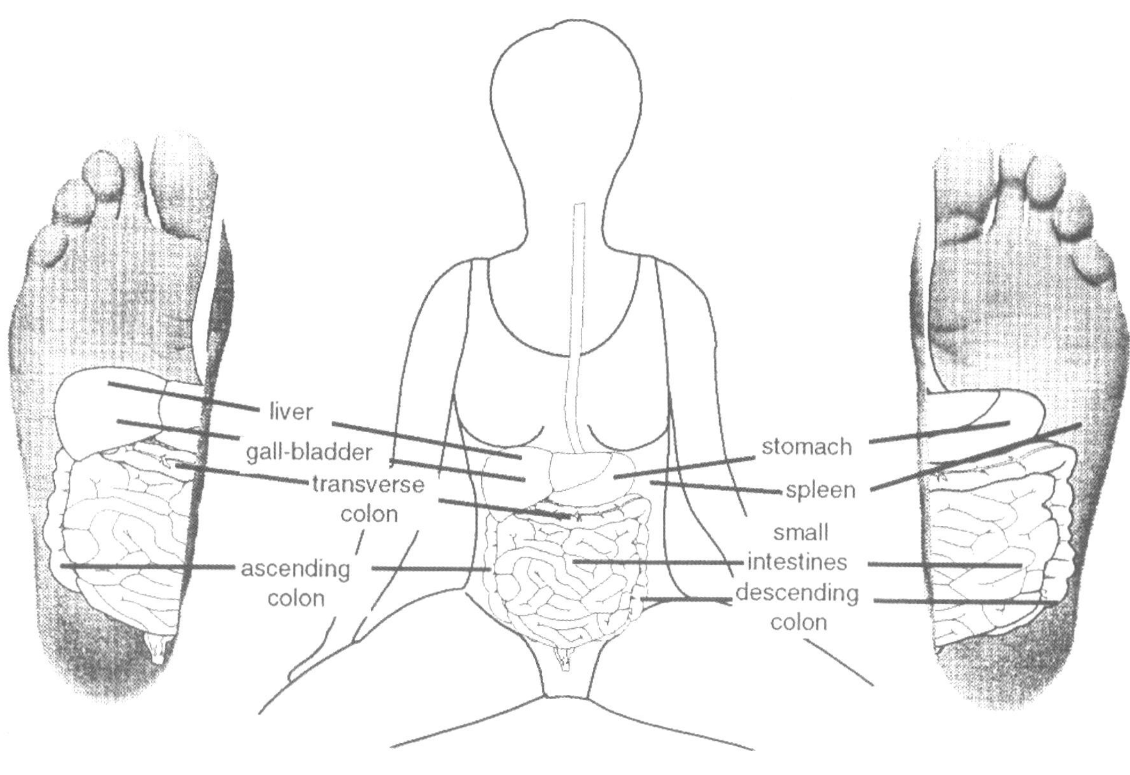

Physiology	During pregnancy the alimentary system does not change; however it has to cope with changed nutritional requirements, food fads and lack of space.
Metaphysical aspects	Metaphysically the alimentary system holds the qualities of ingestion, digestion, absorption, and assimilation of ideas, thoughts and beliefs. The oesophagus holds the ability to swallow concepts - "stuck in the craw". The stomach holds worry, anxiety - "butterflies in the stomach". Small intestines hold misunderstandings, inability to assimilate ideas and dread. Large intestines hold deep gut feelings and guilt. Rectum holds security, terror and "the shits".
Reflexology	Maintain the vitality of the system.

FOOD FADS (PICA)

Food fads are a strong desire to eat unusual foods or bizarre combinations of food at odd times.

Physiology

The body will not allow itself to be poisoned during pregnancy. Some foods that were in the normal diet now become uneatable.

When the body knows that it requires certain substances, for example, minerals, the brain interprets the message and the desire for food containing the substance becomes a "must have".

It is interesting to note that if the fad is imperative then it is the baby's need and if it is less demanding it is the mother's need.

Reflexology

"Balance organ" and "sense of self"	Linking - to remind the client that although she has been taken over by the Incoming Soul she is still herself!
"Solar plexus"	Hold - to ease her anxiety.
Endocrine system	Endocrine balance - to help adjust to the changes.

Extra advice

Reassure the client that food fads are OK. Humour helps with this situation.
If possible encourage her to have good nutrition. This is not always achievable because of morning sickness.

HEARTBURN

Heartburn is a painful burning sensation behind the lower end of the sternum (breast bone).

Physiology

The effect of progesterone relaxes the sphincter between the stomach and oesophagus (gullet) causing reflux of acid stomach contents, which irritates the oesophagus.
Pressure from the growing baby may add to the discomfort.

Caution

DANGER SIGN
A heartburn-like pain (epigastric pain) may be a danger sign for pre-eclampsia. Ensure the client informs her obstetric caregiver.

Reflexology

Stomach	Sedate - to help prevent overactivity.
Oesophagus	Sedate - to ease the pain.
"Solar plexus"	Hold - to calm and relieve anxiety.

Extra advice

- Eat small frequent meals.
- Avoid spicy, fatty or fried foods.
- At meals sit up straight and eat slowly.
- Avoid bending over; squat or kneel instead.
- At night sleep with extra pillows or raise the foot of the bed.

VOMITING - MORNING SICKNESS

Morning sickness is the term used for nausea and vomiting during pregnancy. This is a misnomer as it can be morning, noon and night sickness!

Physiology	The presence of Human Chorionic Gonadotrophin (a pregnancy hormone) is believed to be responsible for morning sickness. Morning sickness occurs more frequently in early pregnancy. High levels of oestrogen can create a heightened sense of smell and aromas can aggravate morning sickness.
Reflexology Stomach	Sedate. Remember she may be "sick" of something or someone.
Pancreas	Gentle stimulation - to improve her "sweetness of life" and help balance her blood sugar levels.
Endocrine system	Endocrine balance - to help her adapt to her changing hormones.
Extra advice	Suggest that she eats small amounts of a food that she can tolerate little and often (about every two hours). Sometimes ginger or peppermint can ease the vomiting.

HYPEREMESIS GRAVIDARUM

Hyperemesis gravidarum is severe and persistent vomiting during pregnancy.

Physiology	Continued vomiting will make the client dehydrated and her electrolytes unbalanced. She will loose weight and stamina.
Caution	**MEDICAL PROBLEM** **This client must see her obstetric caregiver and may need hospitalisation and rehydration.**
Reflexology	As for vomiting.

CONSTIPATION

Constipation is difficult or uncomfortable bowel movements.

Physiology	Progesterone makes the plain muscles relax creating sluggish colon activity. More water is absorbed from the colon making stools harder. Iron tablets can make the situation worse.
Minor Ailment	Some pregnant clients become anxious if they have to strain to have their bowels open.
Reflexology Large intestines	Gentle massage type movements - to encourage bowel activity.
Extra advice	Suggest that the client drinks more water and increases her dietary fibre. Five portions of fruit and/or vegetables is recommended per day.
Caution ⃠	**Omit working the rectum reflex zone during the first trimester.**

DIARRHOEA

Diarrhoea is the passing of many watery or unformed bowel movements.

Physiology	Ingested substances that will harm the body are removed as soon as possible. A prodromal sign of impending labour is to have diarrhoea.
Precaution	If the diarrhoea is severe, ensure the client sees her medical caregiver.

IRRITABLE BOWEL

Irritable bowel may be extreme diarrhoea or a symptom of another disease.

Problem	An irritable bowel can irritate the uterus causing contractions. If it is accompanied by fever it can pre-empt pre-term labour. Dehydration poses a health threat to both mother and baby.
Reflexology Large intestines	Gently rub in the reverse direction of the normal flow - to calm the area.
"Solar plexus"	Hold - to settle the being.
Small intestines	Sedate - to settle the area.
Precaution	Ensure the client sees her medical caregiver.

URINARY SYSTEM

ANATOMICAL PLACEMENT AND REFLEX ZONES

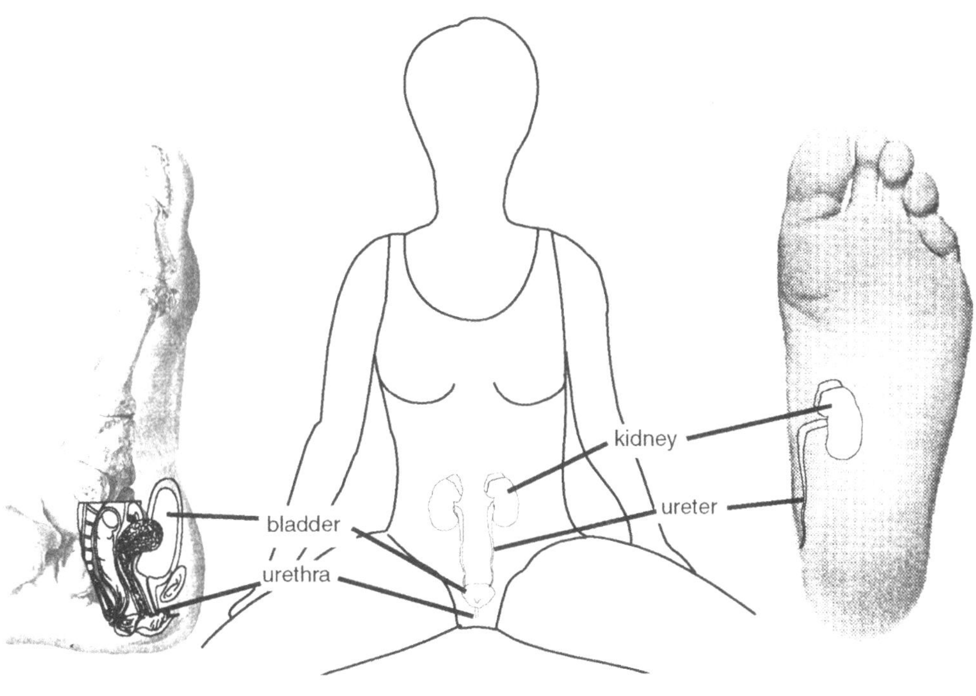

Physiology

During pregnancy the renal threshold is lowered, which means that larger molecules are filtered out. Protein molecules are larger molecules which normally retained are now passed giving the woman mild proteinuria.

The kidneys are particularly vulnerable to the stresses of pregnancy. There is extra fluid (blood and interstitial fluid) in the body that alters the fluid balance requirement.

The kidneys cannot tolerate a sudden rise in blood pressure.

Metaphysical aspects

A concept in the Metamorphic Technique modality is that the fluids of the body have a correspondence with the emotions. The urinary system is one of the fluid systems of the body and demonstrates this concept.

Kidneys hold fear.
The bladder holds frustration and annoyance - "pissed off" feelings.

Reflexology

During pregnancy always treat the kidney reflex zones very gently. Use the urinary system "flush".

FREQUENCY OF MICTURITION

Frequency of micturition is the passing of small amounts of urine frequently.

Physiology

In early pregnancy the normal position of the uterus (anteverted) presses on the bladder causing it to empty frequently. This condition passes as the uterus grows and becomes upright.
At the end of the pregnancy when baby has his head engaged, it presses on the bladder causing it to empty frequently.

Reflexology

Urinary system	"Flush" - to maintain the integrity of the system.
Pelvis	Gentle pelvic relaxation techniques - to relax the area.

In addition

Reassure the client that this is OK.

CYSTITIS / URINARY TRACT INFECTION (UTI)

Cystitis is inflammation or infection of the bladder. UTI is an infection in the urinary system. In addition to frequency of micturition it is characterised by irritation and burning sensation.

Physiology

Frequency of micturition does not cause cystitis.
However for a client who has a history of cystitis the frequency of micturition may be a symptom of cystitis.

MEDICAL PROBLEM

Caution

Cystitis may be a maternal cause of early miscarriage. Ensure the client informs her medical caregiver.

Reflexology

After her obstetric caregiver has checked the client, in addition to the above reflexology include:

Thymus	Tap - to encourage natural immunity.
Lymphatic system	Lymphatic technique - to promote elimination of toxins.

PROTEINURIA

Proteinuria is the presence of protein in the urine. It is detected by routine urinalysis.

MAJOR PROBLEM
Caution

When Proteinuria is associated with oedema and hypertension.
It is a symptom of pre-eclampsia.
Needs obstetric care.

HAEMATURIA

Haematuria is the presence of blood in the urine. It may be detected by urinalysis or may be seen.

MAJOR PROBLEM
Caution

There should never be blood in the urine.
Needs obstetric care.

GLYCOSURIA

Glycosuria is the presence of glucose in the urine. It is detected by routine urinalysis.

MAJOR PROBLEM
Caution

Glycosuria is a symptom of diabetes.
Needs obstetric care.

Note It is not the responsibility of the reflexologist to do the urinalysis.

Reflexology
Urinary system "Flush" - to help maintain health.

CARDIO-VASCULAR SYSTEM

ANATOMICAL PLACEMENT & REFLEX ZONES

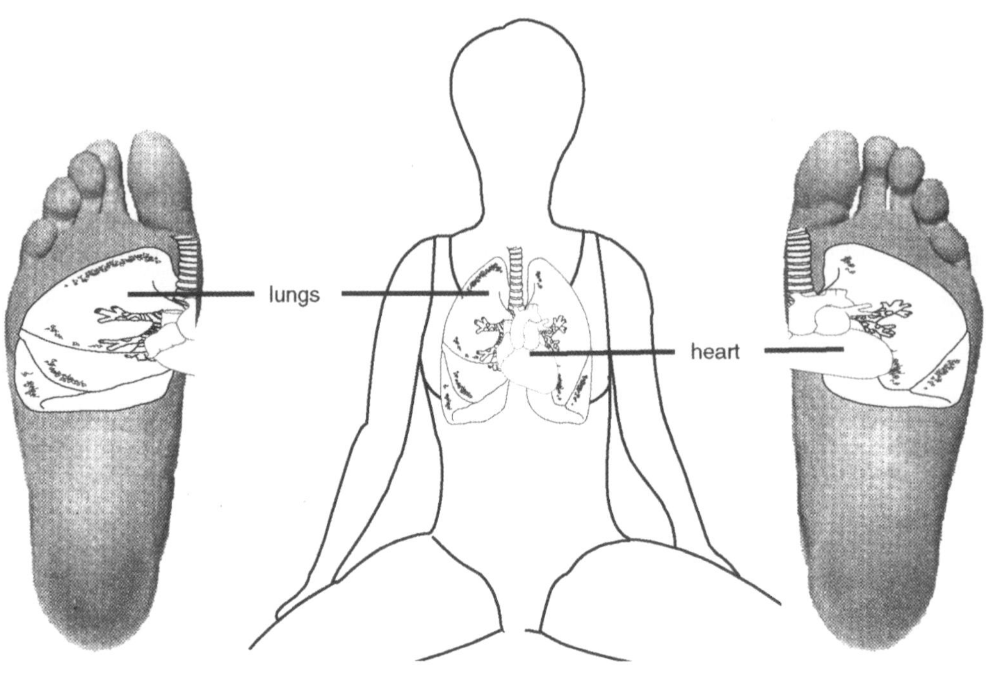

Physiology

The cardio-vascular system undergoes huge changes during pregnancy. The mother's cardiac output has to sustain the placenta and thus the output is increased. There is an increase in the blood volume - hypervolaemia.

Blood pressure is the pressure under which blood is pumped around the body. During pregnancy the blood pressure follows a pattern. The blood pressure is normal for that client during the first trimester, falls slightly during the second trimester and rises again during the third trimester.

Metaphysical aspects

According to Traditional Chinese Medicine (TCM) the heart pumps joy around the body.
According to the Metamorphic Technique modality the effect of the mind and emotions are held in the soft tissues of the body.

The heart holds:

- Love - hate
- Joy - despair
- Courage - cowardice
- Sayings include: "hardening of the heart", "heartache".

Reflexology

Maintain the vitality of the system.

Note

It is not the responsibility of the reflexologist to take the client's blood pressure.

PALPITATIONS

Palpitations are irregular, rapid heartbeats that are noticeable to the client.

Physiology

The increased blood volume (physiological hypervolaemia) in the system makes it possible for the client to feel her heartbeat.

Palpitations are aggravated by inadequate iron level in the blood.

Minor ailment

Palpitations can be worrying but are not dangerous. However if they become too much ensure she informs her medical caregiver.

Reflexology

Chest	Relaxation techniques - to relax and calm.
Heart and "balance organ"	Linking technique - to help regain equilibrium.
"Solar plexus"	Hold - to decrease anxiety.

In addition

This condition may be worrying to the client; reassure her that it is not dangerous.

Explain the physiology - with some understanding it is not so frightening for the client.

CARDIAC CONDITIONS & DISEASES

There are too many cardiac conditions and diseases to enumerate here.

Physiology

One of the effects of hypervolaemia is that doctors can clearly hear cardiac anomalies. Most of them are benign but must be checked by a physician.

MAJOR PROBLEM
Caution

These clients must be in the care of medical and obstetric practitioners.

ANAEMIA

Anaemia is a condition where the oxygen carrying capacity of the blood is decreased due to deficiency in the quality or quantity of red blood cells.

Physiology	During pregnancy blood haemoglobin concentrations drop slightly as the blood volume increases disproportionately to haemoglobin increases. This is known as physiological anaemia.
Minor problem	As pregnancy progresses the condition resolves itself.
Precaution	There are several types of anaemia that can be detrimental to both mother and baby. Ensure the client sees her medical caregiver.

Reflexology

Spleen	Gently stimulate - to encourage red blood cell vitality.
Liver	Gently stimulate - to encourage blood health.
Heart	Gently stimulate - to promote joy.

Extra advice	Suggest the client adapts her diet to include more iron rich foods.

SEVERE ANAEMIA

Severe anaemia may be a symptom of other diseases or a medical condition in itself.

MAJOR PROBLEM	This client must be in the care of obstetric and medical professionals.

VARICOSE VEINS OF THE LEGS

Varicose veins of the legs are veins that become dilated.

Physiology	The veins of the legs have one-way valves to prevent back flow of blood. If the veins are prevented from draining properly the valves may fail. The hormones of pregnancy soften the walls of the veins. As the pregnancy progresses with the weight gain, pressure on the leg veins increases, they swell and may become varicose.
Minor ailment	This condition gets worse as the pregnancy progresses. It continues after the baby is born and deteriorates with each subsequent pregnancy. It is very sore for the mother but does not harm the pregnancy.
Problem	The varicose veins may ulcerate.

Reflexology

Lymphatic system	Lymphatic technique - to improve the vitality of the body.

Extra advice	Remind the client to encourage the blood flow in her legs by not wearing socks with elasticised edges.
Caution	**Do NOT massage the varicose veins.**

CRAMPS IN THE LEGS

Cramps in the legs are muscular spasms that usually occur in the calf muscles.

Physiology	Changes in the blood components: the acid balance, electrolytes, or calcium / salt intake probably cause cramps.
Minor ailment	Cramps in the legs often occur during pregnancy. They are a discomfort but not risky to the pregnancy.
Potential problem	Cramp like pains in the leg may be Deep Vein Thrombosis (DVT). Differentiation between cramps and DVT. It is important to be able to distinguish between leg cramps and (DVT). Dorsiflex the foot. Cramps in the legs welcome dorsiflection. DVT gives a positive Homan's sign.

Reflexology First Aid
Dorsiflex the feet and toes. Advise the client to stamp the balls of her feet with the toes dorsiflexed.

Reflexology

Lymphatic system	Lymphatic technique - to assist removal of toxins.
"Solar plexus"	Hold - to relieve anxiety.
Urinary system	"Flush" - to support the reflexology lymphatic technique.

Caution

Differentiate between cramps and deep vein thrombosis and do NOT use reflexology if in doubt.

DEEP VEIN THROMBOSIS (DVT)

Deep vein thrombosis is a blood clot that forms inside a vein, usually the vein deep in the calf muscle (deep saphenous). It may partially or completely block the blood flow. There is a risk that fragments may detach and travel to another part of the body causing an embolus e.g. pulmonary embolus.

Physiology

High levels of oestrogen and increased blood clotting capability of pregnancy are associated with DVT.

Signs and symptoms

Locally:

- Pain
- Swelling
- Heat
- Redness

Sometimes the client may complain of cramp or there may be no sign at all.

Diagnosis

To test: Dorsiflex the foot.
If there is a DVT there is excruciating pain in the calf - a positive Homan's sign.

Action

DO NOT REPEAT THE TEST

DO NOT MOVE THE CLIENT

SEEK MEDICAL ASSISTANCE IMMEDIATELY

Caution

As reflexology increases the vitality of the vascular system, there is a possibility that the thrombosis may move with dire consequences.

Contraindication

REFLEXOLOGY CONTRAINDICATED

HYPOTENSION

Hypotension is low blood pressure. It can make the woman feel light headed, "swimmy" or faint.

Physiology	Some women naturally have low blood pressure. In some women the pregnancy hormones create this condition.
Minor Ailment	This condition can be a bother to the client but is not dangerous.

SUPINE HYPOTENSION

Supine Hypotension is caused when the client lies down, flat on her back.

Physiology	The weight of the baby presses on the inferior vena cava compressing it and impeding the blood flow to the heart. It frequently occurs during the third trimester of pregnancy.
Preventative measure	Do not let the client lie flat on her back.
Action	If the client is lying on her back roll her onto her side about 5cm, just sufficient for the baby to move off the vein.

POSTURAL HYPOTENSION

Postural Hypotension is caused when the client stands up quickly.

Physiology	The blood pressure is temporally reduced in the brain.
Precaution	This can cause the client to become dizzy and fall.
Action	Sit the client down and advise her to stand up slowly next time.

Reflexology

"Solar plexus"	Gently stimulate - to strengthen the creative energy flow.
Kidneys	Gently stimulate - to increase vitality.
Spine	Spine rub - to increase vitality.

Extra advice	Suggest that when the client is resting she uses pillows to prevent her from rolling on her back. Suggest that she stands up slowly.

HYPERTENSION

Hypertension is raised blood pressure.

Physiology

Some women have pre-existing or essential hypertension.
Increased body weight, blood volume and cardiac output may cause strain on the kidneys resulting in raised blood pressure.

Caution

Hypertension is a potential major obstetric problem.

Reflexology	
Kidneys	Very gently bimanually sedate - to encourage normal function.
Lymphatic system	Lymphatic technique - to assist in the removal of increasing amount of cell debris.
Urinary system	"Flush" - to help the body excrete extra fluid.
"Solar plexus"	Hold - to relieve anxiety and tension.
Adrenal glands	Very gently sedate - to relieve stress.
Diaphragm	Sedate - to ease tension.
Entire body	Relaxation techniques - to settle.

HYPERTENSION ASSOCIATED WITH PROTEINURIA AND OEDEMA

Hypertension associated with proteinuria and oedema are the three main symptoms of pre-eclampsia also known as toxaemia of pregnancy and pregnancy-induced hypertension (PIH). There may be a gradual or sudden onset of this condition.

MAJOR OBSTETRIC PROBLEM

Caution

If untreated pre-eclampsia can develop into fulminating eclampsia which is life threatening to both mother and baby. This client will be in the care of an obstetrician and in hospital.

Danger signs

Danger signs include: frontal headaches, visual disturbances and epigastric pain (a heartburn-like pain).

Precaution

If working with a client with pre-eclampsia obtain written permission from the obstetrician.
Be prepared to work in a darkened room and in silence, as any startle effect is detrimental to the client.

LYMPHATIC SYSTEM

ANATOMICAL PLACEMENT & REFLEX ZONES

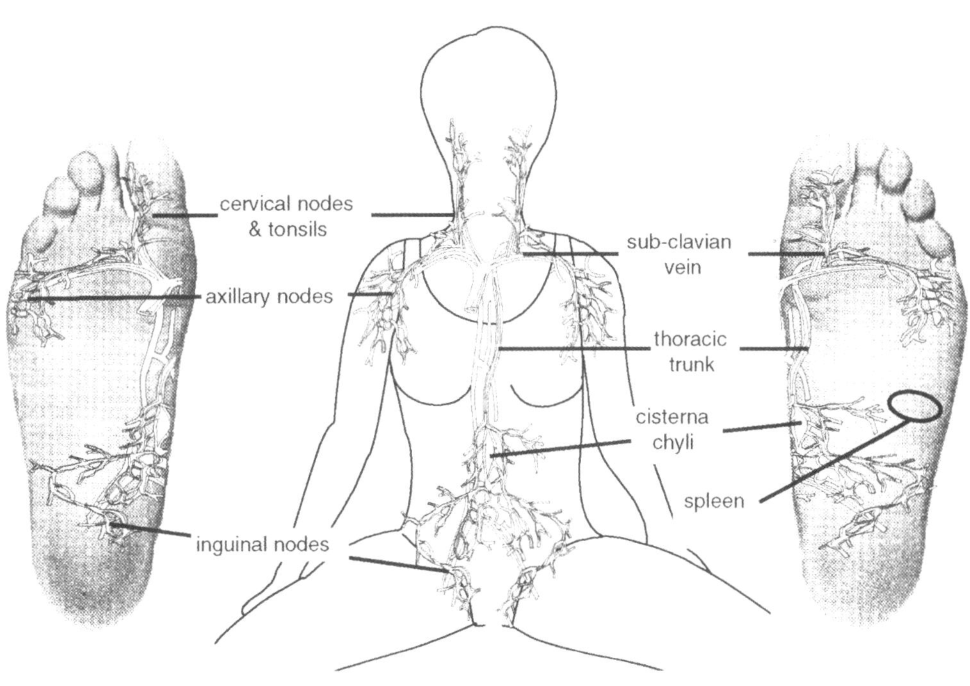

"Babies always make messes" from the time when they are a few cells multiplying until for ever more! During pregnancy the lymphatic system has an extra workload.

Physiology

To cope with the extra workload, that is to remove more cell debris and waste products, most cells retain a small amount of extra fluid and there is an increase in interstitial fluid. This is the body's normal response (physiological oedema). It is necessary and beneficial and recognised as part of the "glow" of good health in pregnancy. The amount of fluid retained increases throughout pregnancy.

Metaphysical aspects

According to the Metamorphic Technique modality the fluids of the body have a correspondence with emotions. When there is oedema present there is a blocking of the movement of fluid and thus the emotions. It is helpful in a reflexology treatment to use this information; it will give greater insight into more ways to support the client.

Reflexology

Use the reflexology lymphatic technique at each session as this maintains the vitality of the lymphatic system.

MODERATE OEDEMA

Moderate oedema is excess interstitial fluid and shows when the client's rings become too tight, when she has ankle oedema or puts on excessive weight.

Physiology

As the pregnancy progresses more fluid is retained especially in hot weather and it is posture aggravated.

Minor ailment

Most clients accept that some oedema is part of pregnancy, but some feel very uncomfortable.

Reflexology

Lymphatic system — Lymphatic technique - to persuade the body to remove excess fluid. It may be necessary to repeat this technique several times.

Urinary system — Extremely gentle "flush - to help maintain fluid balance.

"Solar plexus" — Hold - to support life force.

Remember to use the knowledge of the fluid correspondences.

Extra advice

Advise the client to remove her rings as they may become too tight.

SEVERE OEDEMA

Severe oedema shows when the client's body looks "water logged". The client's eyes may look as though she has "unshed tears".

Physiology

The body retains an excess of fluid, probably to assist the removal of toxins or other waste matter that has accumulated.

POTENTIAL MAJOR PROBLEM
Caution

This is a potential major obstetric problem, client must have obstetric care. Danger signs include frontal headaches, blurred vision and visual disturbances and heartburn-like sensations.

SEVERE OEDEMA ASSOCIATED WITH HYPERTENSION AND PROTEINURIA

Severe oedema when associated with hypertension and proteinuria are the symptoms of pre-eclampsia also known as toxaemia of pregnancy or pregnancy-induced hypertension (PIH). If untreated fulminating eclampsia can develop which is life threatening to both mother and baby.

MAJOR OBSTETRIC PROBLEM
Caution

Major obstetric problem and essential to have obstetric care.

Physiology

Kidney function may be compromised and the fluid balance affected.

Precaution

To use reflexology with these clients the prime obstetric caregiver must prescribe it. Work very gently in silence in a darkened room.

Reflexology

If it is prescribed by the obstetric caregiver reflexology lymphatic technique can complement the medical treatment to help prevent eclampsia.

RESPIRATORY SYSTEM

ANATOMICAL PLACEMENT & REFLEX ZONES

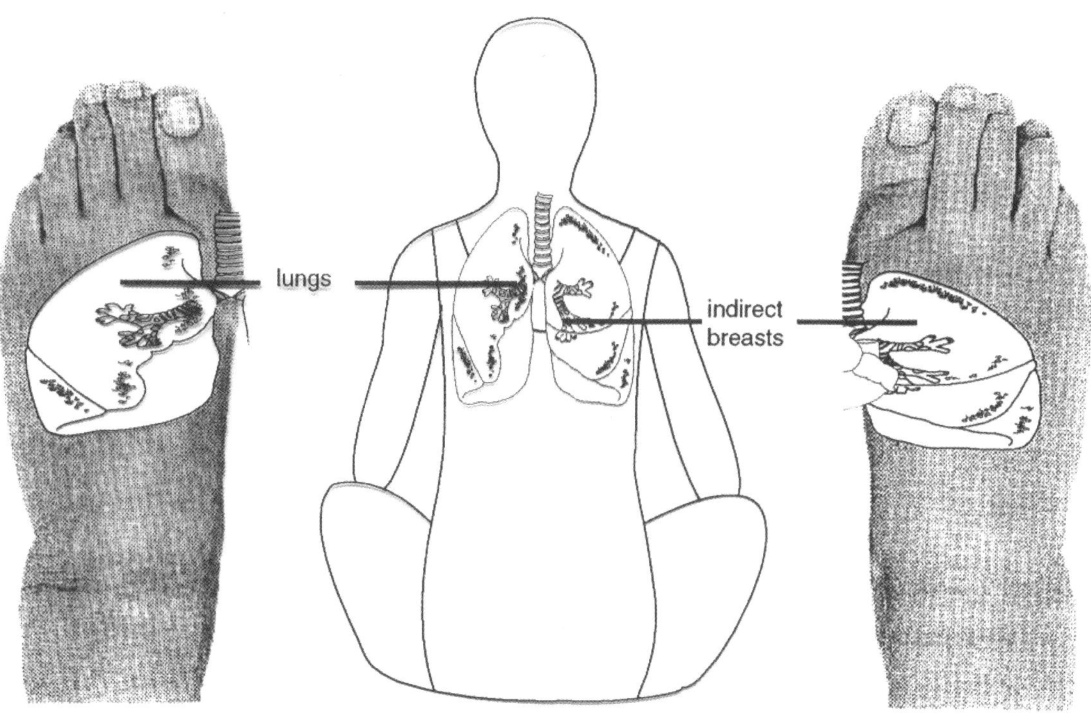

Physiology

During pregnancy the respiratory system is subject to extensive changes. The shape of the chest alters to increase the lung capacity by flaring the lower ribs. The respiratory system is susceptible to the emotions. Towards the end of pregnancy it is susceptible to abdominal pressure.

Metaphysical aspects

The respiratory system deals with the animation principle of air.
Breath means life, the ability to take in life.
Breath is direct contact between self and the world.
Breathing = exchange:

- Giving - taking
- Contracting - relaxing
- In - out

Vital to life - imagine how long a person can live without food, how long without water and how long without air.

Note

Lungs hold: unhappiness, sadness and grief.
Throat is an avenue of expression, a channel of creativity.
With a newborn baby's first breath he is independent and free.

Reflexology

Maintain the vitality of the system.

PANIC ATTACKS

Panic attacks are times of sudden alarm or fright that can be unreasoning or excessive.

Physiology

The hormones of pregnancy keep the mother's sense of preservation of the next generation instantly available. Adrenaline cuts in and she responds immediately.
The mother's emotions are more labile during pregnancy and things that would not normally upset her now do so.

Minor problem

This is yet another thing that can happen during pregnancy. If it occurs frequently the client would be well advised to seek counselling.

HYPERVENTILATION

Hyperventilation is over breathing. The respirations are often rapid and shallow.

Physiology

Rapid respirations cause the carbon dioxide levels in the blood to decrease, temporarily upsetting the normal blood chemistry.
The client can feel dizzy and even faint.

Problem

As the baby gets his oxygen from his mother he needs a constant steady supply.

Reflexology First Aid

"Solar plexus"	Hold - to calm and settle.
Shoulder girdle	Relaxation techniques - to ease tension.
Lungs	Lung press - to regulate respirations.

Extra advice

Wherever possible avoid anxiety-producing situations, stress and fatigue.

Use the brown paper bag trick:

- Cover the mouth and nose with a brown paper bag (or cupped hands)
- Slowly breathe out into the bag
- Re-breathe in the air from the bag
- Repeat about ten times.

Learn some breathing techniques to use as a coping strategy.

NERVOUS SYSTEMS

ANATOMICAL PLACEMENT & REFLEX ZONES

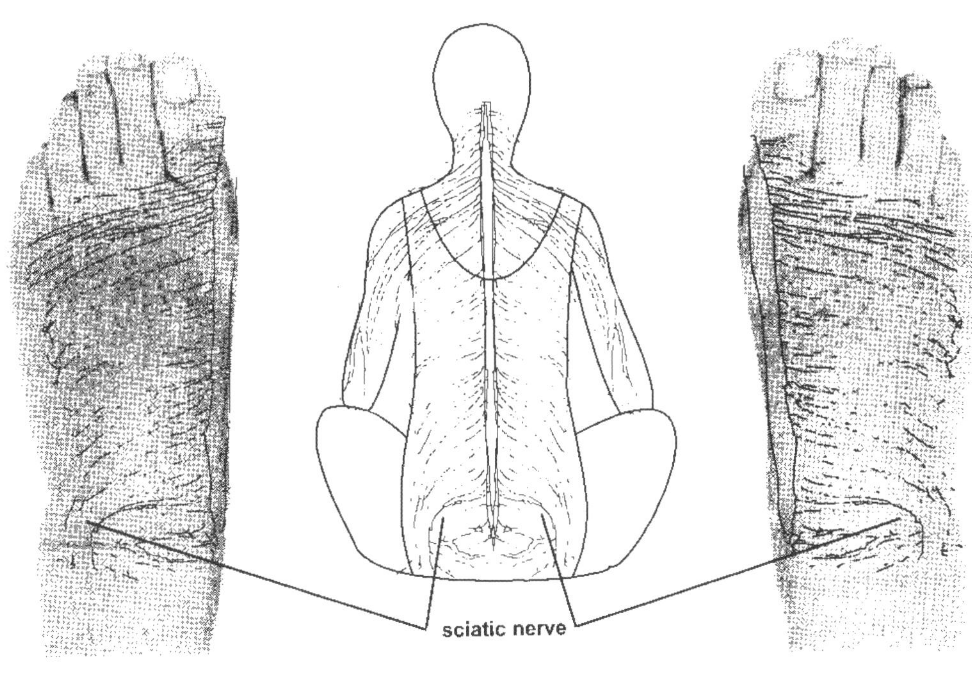

Physiology	The nervous systems are influenced by physical changes in the body.
Metaphysical aspects	The nervous systems are part of the animation of the body. Animation includes nerve impulses and the senses and is an almost indefinable interaction between body, mind and soul. Animation is the energy that maintains life force.
Reflexology	Maintain the health of the systems.

CARPAL TUNNEL SYNDROME

Carpal tunnel syndrome is a condition that results from compression of the median nerve in the carpal tunnel of the wrist.

Physiology	Fluid retention may cause the tissues in the wrist to become oedematous and encroach on the carpal tunnel of the wrist making the hand and wrist weak and clumsy and causing pain.
Minor ailment	This condition is uncomfortable / debilitating, and makes the hand and fingers clumsy. However it is not a threat to the pregnancy.
Reflexology	
Wrist, referral areas	Sedate the referral areas of the affected wrist - to ease pain.
Lymphatic system	Lymphatic technique - to lessen oedema.
Urinary system	"Flush" - to help balance fluid levels and promote excretion of urine.
"Solar plexus"	Hold - to ease anxiety.
Extra advice	An old fashioned warm poultice applied to the affected wrist is very soothing

SCIATICA

Sciatica is a painful condition resulting from irritation of the sciatic nerve.

Physiology	The pregnancy hormone relaxin increases laxity of the ligaments and the altered posture caused by the pregnancy narrows the holes through which the sciatic nerves pass thus nipping them.
Minor ailment	This condition can be anything from mildly uncomfortable to devastatingly painful. It is very unpleasant for the mother but does not affect the pregnancy.
Extra advice	Suggest that the client consults an osteopath who works with pregnant women.
Reflexology First Aid	
Greater sciatic foramen	Trigger Point Release - to release trapped energy.
Caution	**The Trigger Point Release technique is not suitable for most reflex zones during pregnancy. This is one exception**
Reflexology	
Hip and pelvis	Gentle relaxation techniques - to relax the area.
Spine	Pregnancy adapted spinal twist - to encourage movement.
"Solar plexus"	Hold - to relieve anxiety.
Extra advice	Alternate warm and cold packs over the painful area - to increase tissue-repairing ability.

HEADACHES

Headaches are pains in the head. They may be in one specific area or generally all over the head.

Physiology	Changes in the hormone levels give a different body environment. Increased blood volume (hypervolaemia) may increase the pressure in the head. Tension and anxiety may tighten the neck muscles. The weather, especially hot and stormy, affects pregnant women. A rising blood pressure will cause headaches.
Minor ailment	This condition is often considered yet another of the minor ailments of pregnancy.
Reflexology	
Head and neck	Toe rotations and stretches - to relax the head and neck.
Spine	Gentle pregnancy adapted spinal twists - to relax back tension and release energy flow.
Diaphragm	Relaxations to release emotional energy.
Extra advice	A cool footbath is often good for a hot head.
MAJOR PROBLEM **Caution**	**A frontal headache may be a sign of rising blood pressure.** **Ensure the client informs her obstetric caregiver IMMEDIATELY.**

VISUAL DISTURBANCES

Visual disturbances include seeing "floaters", sparkles/lights, shapes and shadows that are not there, "holes" in the vision

MAJOR PROBLEM **Caution**	**Visual disturbances, combined with a frontal headache are signs of rising blood pressure.** **Ensure the client informs her obstetric caregiver IMMEDIATELY.**

MAMMARY AND INTEGUMENTARY SYSTEMS

ANATOMICAL PLACEMENT & REFLEX ZONES

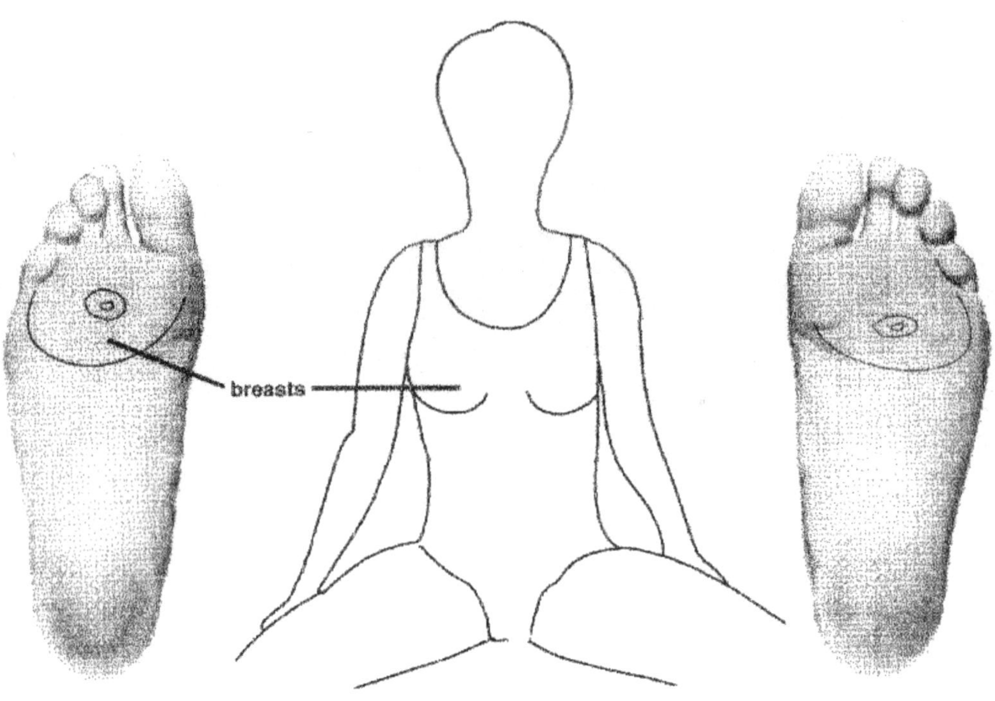

Physiology	**Breasts:** Maximum development of the breasts occurs during pregnancy. Breast changes are one of the first signs of pregnancy. Small raised spots appear around the nipple - Montgomery's tubercles. These tubercles become more prominent and secrete sebum to keep the nipple soft and supple. Nipple size and pigmentation increase during the initial months of pregnancy. As pregnancy progresses blood flow to the breast increases showing as surface veins. More mammary tissue is created increasing the size of the breasts. From about sixteen weeks gestation the breasts prepare for breast-feeding by making colostrum. **Skin:** Changes of colour occur on the skin: nipples darken, a brown line from the pubic bone to the umbilicus (linea nigra) and sometimes a blotchy face or the "mask of pregnancy" (Chloasma). The skin of the breasts, abdomen and thighs and buttocks is stretched.
Metaphysical aspects	The **breasts** are the organs of nurturing. The **integumentary system** (the skin) is the façade that people show to the world. The skin protects our individuality. Sayings: "Get under ones skin", "skin deep", "no skin off my nose".
Reflexology	Maintain the health of the systems.

TENDER BREASTS

Tender breasts are one of the first signs of pregnancy. There is often a prickling / tingling sensation during the early weeks of pregnancy. The increased level of sensation is often replaced by discomfort or pain at about six to eight weeks gestation.

Physiology	The rapid growth of mammary tissue can cause discomfort or pain.
Minor ailment	This is considered a minor ailment and many women and their partners enjoy the increased breast size.
Problem	If the pain is severe ensure the client informs her obstetric caregiver.

Reflexology	
Breasts	Thumb walking and massage type movements - to promote growth and change and to encourage free flow of love energy.

ITCHY SKIN / STRETCH MARKS

Itchy skin commonly occurs on the thighs, breasts and abdomen during late pregnancy. It usually precedes stretch marks.

Physiology	A rapid increase in growth causes the lower layers of the skin to split causing itchiness and stretch marks.
Minor ailment	This condition is fairly common in pregnancy. It can be distressing to the client but does not affect the pregnancy.
MAJOR PROBLEM	Extreme itchiness. See Cholestasis below.

Reflexology

Endocrine system	Balance - to endeavour to prevent stretch marks..
Lymphatic system	Lymphatic technique - to help prevention of accumulation of bile salts
Urinary system	"Flush" - to promote the excretion of urine.
Liver and gall bladder	Gently stimulate- to encourage normal function.

Extra advice	Nothing is guaranteed to prevent stretch marks. However some aromatherapists who are qualified to work with pregnant clients can create lovely preparations to ease the condition.

CHOLESTASIS

Cholestasis is a problem characterised by an accumulation of bile salts. The skin becomes intensely irritating. The irritation is worse at night. The client may try to ease the itching by scratching so much that she causes her palms and soles to bleed.

Physiology	An accumulation of bile salts causes the irritation.
MAJOR OBSTETRIC PROBLEM **Caution**	**Cholestasis is thought to be a cause of late foetal death. Ensure the client informs her obstetric caregiver.**

ENDOCRINE SYSTEM

ANATOMICAL PLACEMENT & REFLEX ZONES

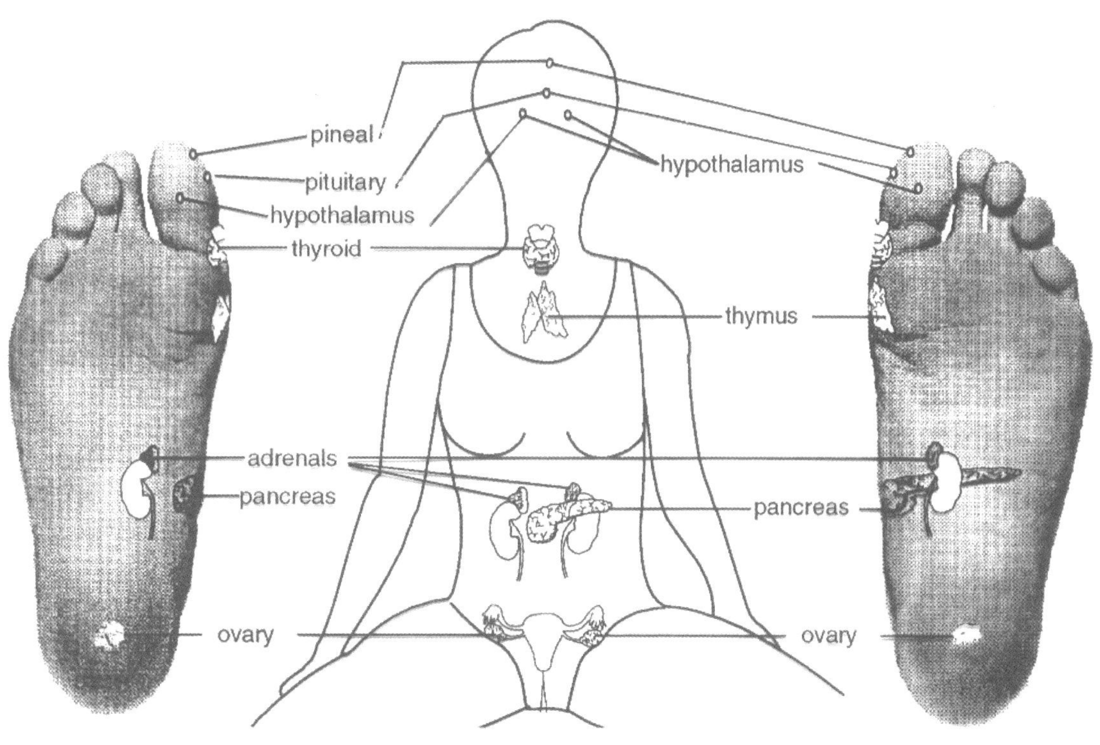

Physical aspect

The **first trimester of pregnancy** is dominated by the hormone Human Chorionic Gonadotrophin (HCG). Its function is to maintain the pregnancy until the placenta is well established.

In the **second trimester of pregnancy** the placenta is established. The function of the placental hormones is to produce and maintain a healthy pregnancy with both mother and baby growing and developing at a steady rate.

In the **third trimester of pregnancy** the output of all the hormones increase. They include: Human Somatomammotropin (HCS), prolactin, relaxin, oestrogen and progesterone.

At the end of pregnancy before birthing commences progesterone levels diminish.

Metaphysical aspect

Spiritual energy enters the body through the seven major chakras. At each point of entry an endocrine gland converts the spiritual energy into physical energy (hormones - the body's chemical messengers).

The Incoming Soul influences the entire hormonal development during pregnancy.

Reflexology

Use an endocrine balance with each treatment. With the enormous normal changing levels of hormones during pregnancy this will balance the client at all stages of her pregnancy.

FATIGUE

Fatigue is a state of being tired and weary.

Physiology	In early pregnancy the effect of the hormone Human Chorionic Gonadotrophin (HCG) and presence of the Incoming Soul cause fatigue. During the last few weeks of pregnancy sleep disturbance, increased weight and day-to-day activities can be tiring.
Minor ailment	Pregnancy makes physical and emotional demands on a woman. Sometimes her lifestyle and activities need to adapt to her status.
Problem	If the fatigue becomes debilitating ensure the client informs her medical caregiver. Fatigue may be a symptom of disease.
Reflexology	
Endocrine system	Balance - to balance the being to the rapidly changing hormone levels.
Spleen	Gentle stimulation - to encourage the production of red blood cells.
"Solar plexus"	Hold - to support the extra demand on life energy.
Longitudinal zones	"Brazilian toe balance" - to balance body energies.
"Balance organ" and hypothalamus	Linking technique - to balance and allow sleep to happen.
Extra advice	Reassure the client that fatigue is a normal reaction to pregnancy.

DIABETES

Diabetes is a disease of the metabolism characterised by the inability of the body to produce enough insulin to process carbohydrates, fats and protein efficiently.

GESTATIONAL DIABETES

Gestational diabetes is diabetes that occurs during pregnancy.

Physiology	During pregnancy a woman's carbohydrate metabolism changes to make glucose more readily available. The pancreas produces more insulin to cope with this glucose. The extra demands for insulin cannot always be met, resulting in sugar intolerance.
MAJOR PROBLEM **Caution**	**This is already a major obstetric problem.** **The client must be in the care of both obstetrician and endocrinologist. Her pregnancy will be closely monitored.** **Once the baby is born a paediatrician will be needed to check him as he may have problems resulting from his mother's diabetes.**
Note	Nowadays diabetic women have better control over their disease and their pregnancies are much safer for themselves, their babies and their diabetes.
Reflexology Endocrine system	Balance - to balance the being to the rapidly changing hormone levels.
Caution	**The energies of reflexology will endeavour to balance the client's glucose level with the result that after a treatment she may have more insulin in her body than it needs at the time, causing her to become hypoglycaemic.**
Caution	**Ensure that the client checks her blood sugar levels BEFORE she leaves your care. If necessary use first aid for the "hypo" (jelly babies).**
Note	**It is NOT the responsibility of the reflexologist to do blood sugar tests.**

PSYCHOLOGICAL ASPECTS

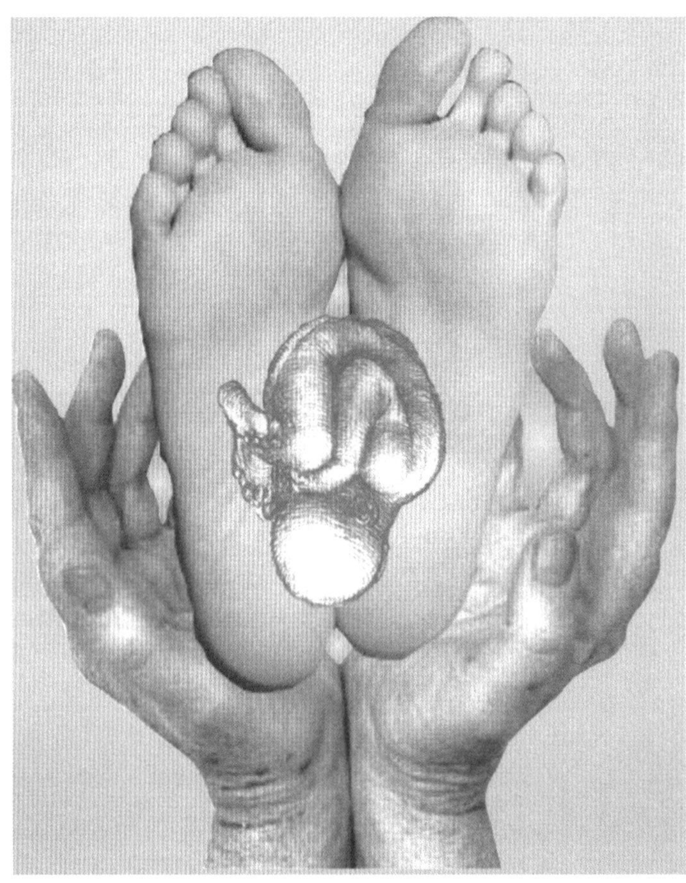

Physiology	Every physical change creates a psychological response and in addition the woman lives with the everyday miracle of the Incoming Soul. There may be fears and anxieties. During pregnancy the woman's emotional state is different from her non-pregnant state. As pregnancy progresses calm women may become more "neurotic", anxious women may become more relaxed, timid women may become more confident and self-assured women may become tentative.
Metaphysical aspects	Everyday Miracle of the The Incoming Soul
Reflexology	The emphasis of care during pregnancy tends to be mainly on the physical aspects and the feelings and emotions of the client can often be ignored. Exceptional care is given by the reflexologist with skills to appreciate the psychology when the client is experiencing one of the most momentous times in her life.

MOOD SWINGS

Mood swings are feelings and emotions that range from happy to miserable, laughing to tears with no apparent rhyme or reason.

Reproduction is a miracle. During this special time the pregnant woman needs to be nurtured and cherished. Lethargy and mood swings caused by hormone changes provide reminders of the effort her body is making to ensure optimum conditions for the development of her baby. The pregnant woman may need to be reminded not to feel guilty or inadequate if she does not maintain her life style as well as nurturing her baby.

Physiology	Increasing amounts of hormones create labile emotions. The Incoming Soul within her puts the woman's sensitivity and intuition on "high voltage". She is naturally more emotional than in her non-pregnant state.
Minor ailments	Some people perceive the heightened emotional response to be a minor ailment.
Precaution **Potential problem**	When the mood swings are too severe or aggravated by stress or become too despairing the client needs extra support such as counselling or some form of coping skills.

Reflexology

Endocrine system	Balance - to help adjust to the huge changes of pregnancy.
"Solar plexus"	Hold - to centre and calm and allow the energy of creation to flow.
"Balance organ" and "sense of self"	Link - to restore "sense of self".

INSOMNIA

Insomnia is failure to get a good night's sleep, including failure to get to sleep and failure to stay asleep.

Physiology	Nocturnal frequency of micturition, excitement, nervousness, tension, anxiety, physical discomfort and an active baby all can cause lack of sleep and an inability to fall asleep.
Minor ailment	The lack of sleep at the end of pregnancy is as though Mother Nature is preparing the mother-to-be for the next year when she will miss out on a lot of sleep.
Problem	The client can become sleep deprived and be unable to cope. Ensure the client informs her obstetric caregiver.

Reflexology

Entire body	All relaxation techniques - to encourage restfulness and tranquillity.
"Solar plexus"	Hold - to settle and calm.
Chest and lung	Breathing techniques - to steady respirations.
Heart	Sedate - to settle the spirit.
Head	Toe stretches and rotations - to calm the mind.
"Balance organ" and hypothalamus	Linking technique - to balance body and mind.

Note	The client may not sleep longer but she will have quality sleep.

Reflexology Techniques

REFLEXOLOGY LYMPHATIC TECHNIQUE

GENERAL INFORMATION

The lymphatic system

The lymphatic system is working to its capacity during pregnancy. It is important to maintain its vitality.

Effects of pregnancy

The effects of pregnancy, hormones, weather and increasing weight gain all take their toll on the client's lymphatic system.

Benefits

Benefits of the reflexology lymphatic technique are that it is not only pleasurable to give and receive, but also an effective way to maintain good health.

Uses

The uses of the technique are:

- To support the vitality of the lymphatic system.
- To support fluid balance.
- To help move toxins and impurities.

Midwives

Midwives who use the technique are finding that oedema associated with hypertension is lessened, the clients feel more comfortable and their blood pressure is more stable.

Research project

A research project undertaken by midwives at Gosford Hospital, NSW, Australia shows a *"significant statistical change"* in the clients who were given the reflexology lymphatic technique.

SPECIFIC INFORMATION

Massage technique

The reflexology lymphatic technique uses a massage style movement and massage oil.

Carrier oil

Use a cold pressed vegetable oil such as sweet almond or grape seed oil.

Precaution - Allergy

Check that the client does not have an allergy or sensitivity to the oil.

Caution - Essential oils

Although the public can buy and use essential oils, unless trained to do so the reflexologist may not use them on clients.

End of session

Because massage oil is used it is suggested to do the reflexology lymphatic technique at the end of a reflexology session.

TECHNIQUES

Movement of lymph reflected

This special technique reflects the movement of the lymphatic system through the body. Interstitial fluid moves from the cells into the lymphatic capillaries, then to the lymphatic veins and trunks and is returned to the circulatory system at the subclavian veins.

"Squidge"

A massage-type technique is used - the movement being similar to squeezing toothpaste up from the bottom of the tube. In this text it is called "squidge".

"Dump"

The movement terminating the "squidge" is like a firm press / prod. In this text it is called "dump".

The aim

The aim of this technique is to clear one area, fill it up then re-clear it, all the time working from the extremities to the centre then to the subclavian vein reflex zone.

Method

Repeat each movement three or four times.

Speed & pressure

Adapt the speed of the movements and the pressure used to the client's need.
For healthy clients use fairly stimulating movements.
For delicate clients or those who like it slow and sensuous use deliberate movements.
For clients with ankle oedema, use very gentle pressure and slow movements.

How often?

Use the technique at each reflexology session.
Repeat it as often as desired.

Note

For clients with ankle oedema the author has used this technique throughout the entire reflexology session, to the exclusion of other reflexology techniques.

EXPECTED OUTCOME

Expected outcome

The expected outcome for using this technique is a diuresis, that is, the client can expect to pass urine fairly soon after.

If the client has oedematous feet and ankles, her feet will feel less tense and her shoes will be more comfortable.

Precaution

If the client has a medical problem for instance cardiac or renal impairment, ensure that you have the medical caregiver's permission to carry out this technique.

THE ROUTINE

Method

Begin with the plantar aspect of the left foot

		REFLEX ZONE	MOVEMENT
1	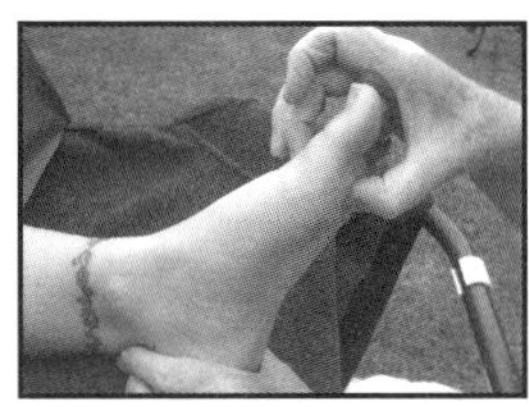	Subclavian vein	Use thumb and index finger, pinch / pump through the foot.
2	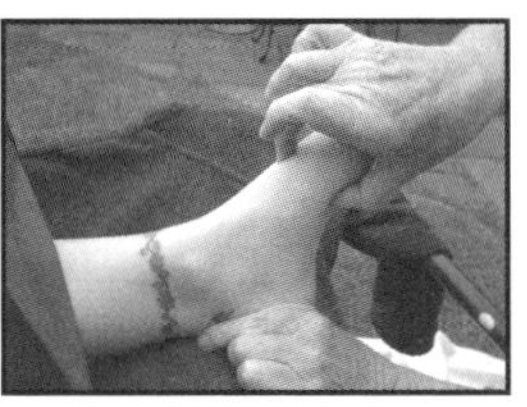	Direct and indirect thoracic trunk and abdominal cysterna chyli	With thumb and index finger both sides of the foot use a pinching and milking type movement. Begin each movement increasingly further away from the subclavian vein reflex zone and end it at the subclavian vein with a pinch.
3	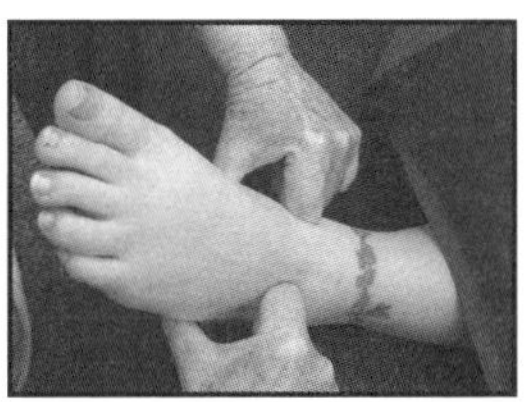	"Eyes of the ankle"	Use index finger knuckles - press into zones.
4	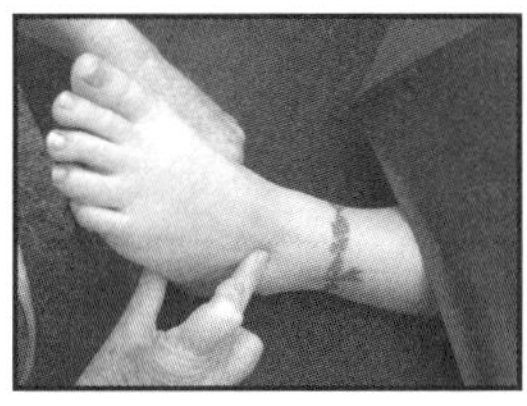	Lower back lymphatics	Squidge from lateral to medial "eye of ankle".
5	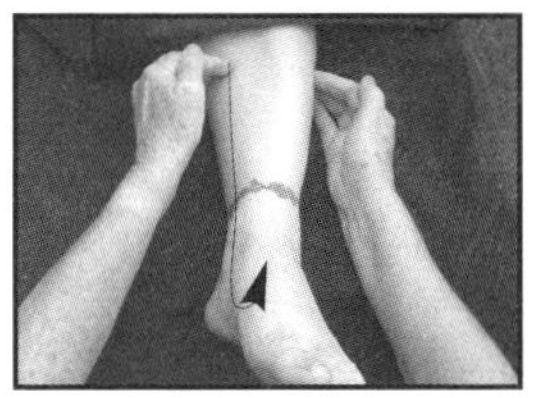	"Chronic" pelvic area	Use all eight fingers - drag from about mid-way up both sides of the leg, around the hips and pelvis and dump into "eyes of the ankle".
6		Repeat 4	
7	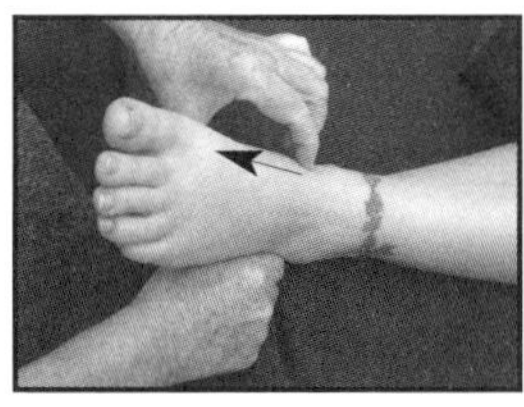	Indirect abdominal cysterna chyli	Squidge from medial "eye of ankle" to waist line.

	REFLEX ZONE	MOVEMENT
8	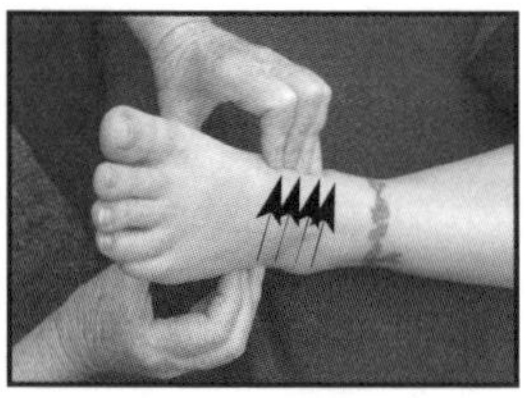 Lower back lymphatics	Use four fingers squidge from the sides of the foot and dump into abdominal chyli cysterna.
9	Repeat 7	
10	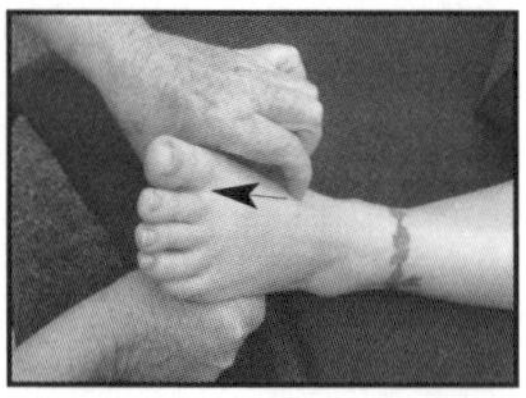 Indirect thoracic trunk	Squidge from waist line, dump into subclavian vein.
11	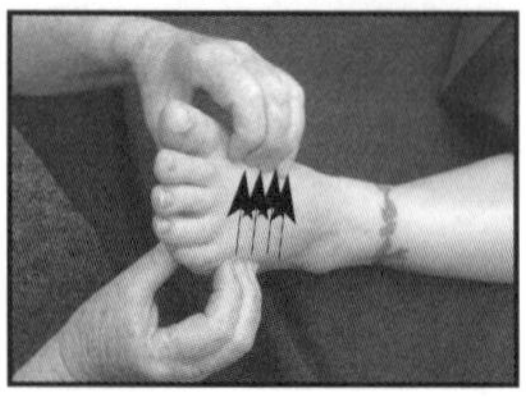 Upper back lymphatics	Use four fingers squidge from the sides of the foot and dump into thoracic trunk.
12	Repeat 7	
13	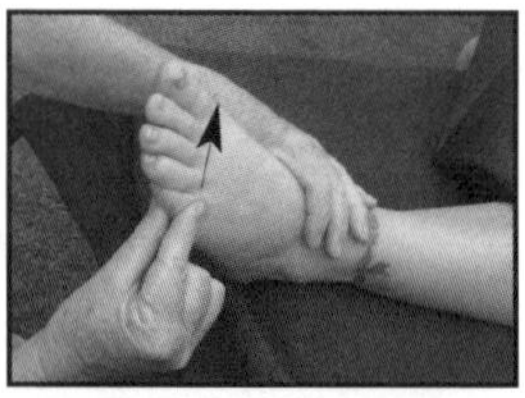 Shoulder lymphatics	Use thumb and index finger, squidge from lateral to medial and dump into subclavian vein.
14	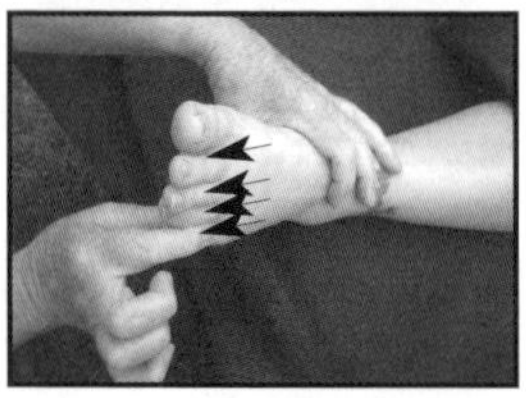 Neck lymphatics	Use thumb and index finger pinch the webbing between each toe in turn and drag from the dorsum of the foot to the plantar aspect.
15	Repeat 13	
16	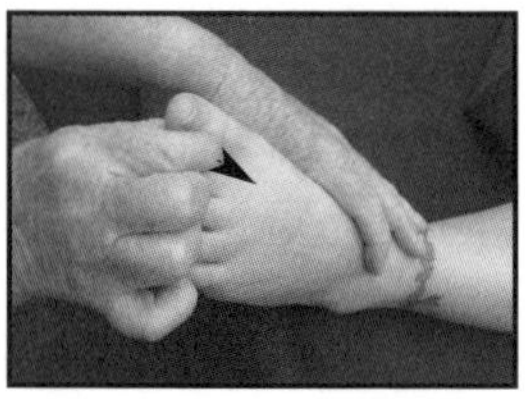 Throat lymphatics	Use thumb or index finger Squidge from below the ear, dump into subclavian vein.

Method

Continue on the plantar aspect of the left foot

		REFLEX ZONE	MOVEMENT
1	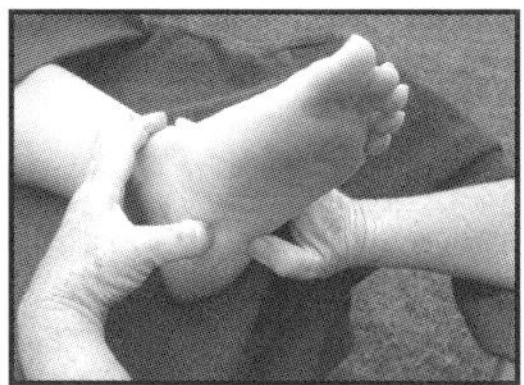	Inguinal nodes	Use both thumbs, press / pump.
2	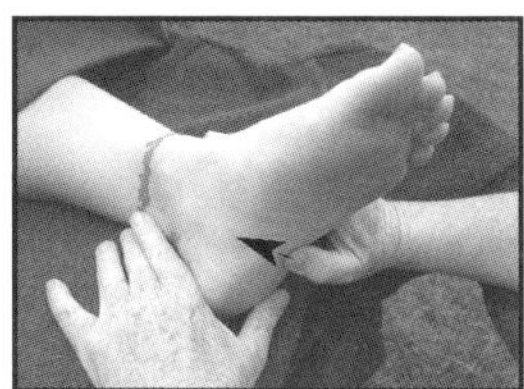	Groin	Squidge from lateral to medial inguinal node.
3	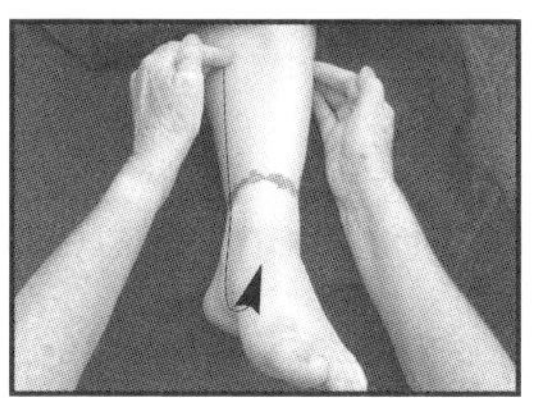	"Chronic" pelvic area	Use all eight fingers - drag from about mid-way up both sides of the leg, across the hips and pelvis and dump into inguinal nodes.
4		Repeat 2	
5	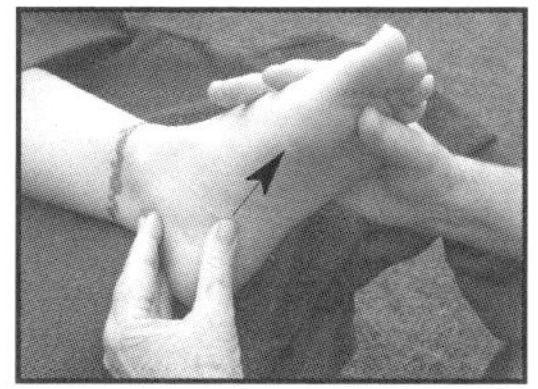	Abdominal cysterna chyli	Use thumb, squidge from medial inguinal node to diaphragm.
6	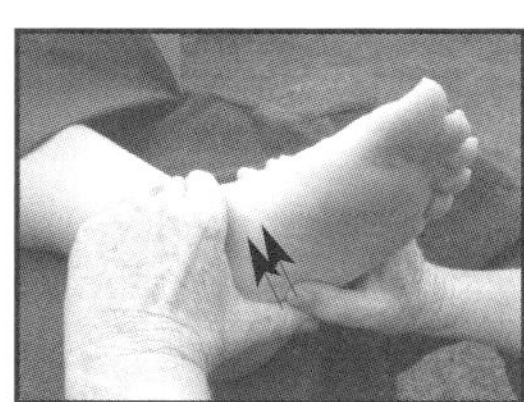	Abdominal lymphatics	Use both thumbs, squidge from lateral to medial, dump into abdominal chyli cysterna.
7		Repeat 5	
8	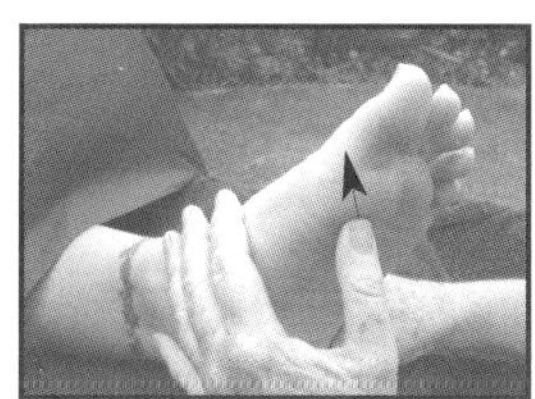	Thoracic trunk	Use thumb, squidge from diaphragm dump into subclavian vein.

	REFLEX ZONE	MOVEMENT
9	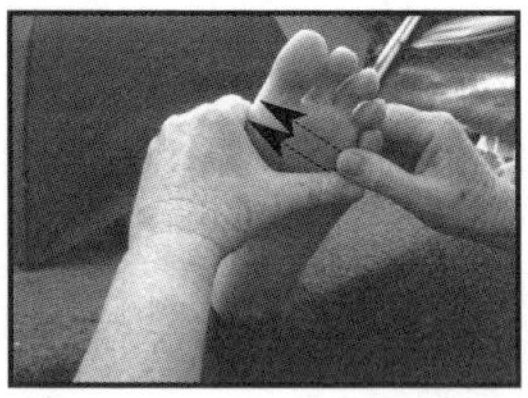 Breast and chest lymphatics	Use both thumbs, squidge from lateral to medial, dump into thoracic trunk.
10	Repeat 8	
11	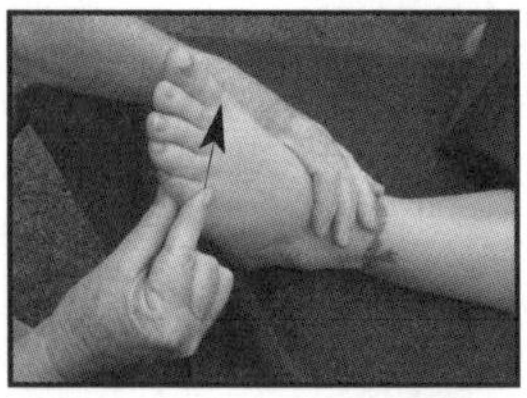 Shoulder lymphatics	Use thumb and index finger, squidge from lateral to medial and dump into subclavian vein.
12	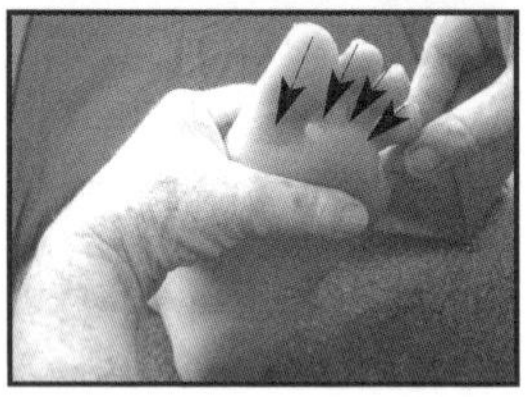 Sinuses and head lymphatics	Use the fingers and thumb of one hand, begin with the little toe, squidge sinus and head, dump into shoulder lymphatics.
13	Repeat 11	
14	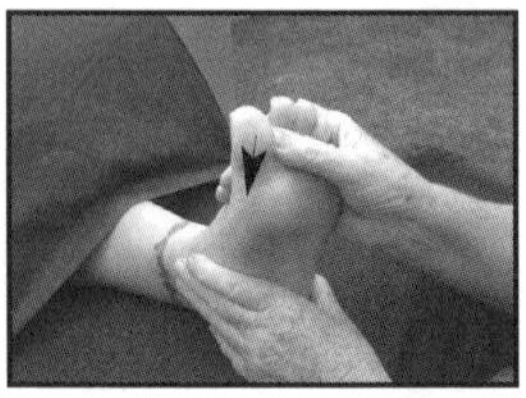 Throat lymphatics	Use thumb or index finger Squidge from below the ear, dump into subclavian vein.
15	Repeat from 1 to 14 on right foot.	
16	Urinary system flush.	

Part 4: The Incoming Soul & Pregnant Feet

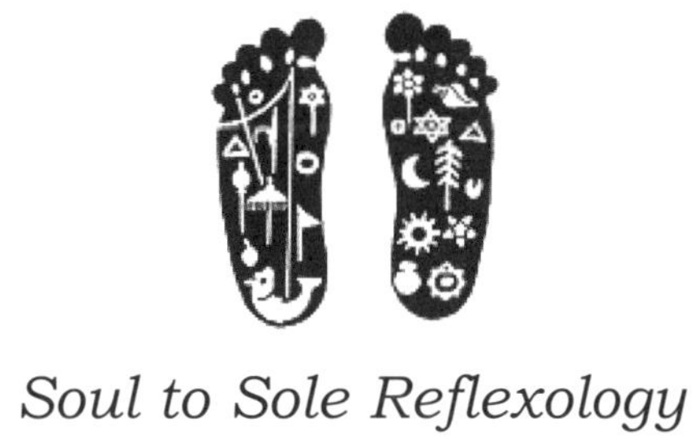

Soul to Sole Reflexology

Introduction to the Incoming Soul and Pregnant Feet

A concept of reflexology is that everything in the being has a reflexion in the feet, The Incoming Soul is no exception. One of the thrilling experiences about Maternity Reflexology is to sense the energy of the Incoming Soul on the feet of the mother.

The Incoming Soul

Here the term "Incoming Soul" is used to identify the entity that is:

- A spiritual energy with an intention of experiencing a human existence.
- A collection of cells.
- An embryo.
- A foetus.
- A baby.

Miracle

The absolute miracle of this every-day occurrence is awesome.

Belief system

Most people have their own belief system about the spiritual realm. The author acknowledges all beliefs and in this text assumes that there is a spiritual state.

Pregnant feet

Naturally the miracle of pregnancy is reflected in the feet of the mother.

RELATED MODALITY

The Metamorphic Technique

The Metamorphic Technique is a modality that has been developed by Gaston Saint-Pierre from a system of Metamorphosis created by Robert St John an Australian reflexologist.
The Metamorphic Technique is a wide-ranging, comprehensive modality and part of it includes the "Prenatal Pattern".

The Prenatal Pattern

While creating Metamorphosis Robert St John observed that the pattern of the reflex of the gestation period is recorded on the spine reflex zones. The author feels that this is of great significance to maternity reflexologists. When working with pregnant clients it is important to be aware of the metaphysical development of the Incoming Soul.

Recommended reading

The Metamorphic Technique, by Gaston Saint-Pierre and Debbie Shapiro.

Foetal experience

"The area of the foot corresponding to the spinal cord, representing the period of gestation generally corresponds with chronic patterns to be identified on the foot in the same transverse strip. A connection exists between foetal experience and postnatal events."
(Avi Grinberg)

On following pages the author has combined the physical and metaphysical aspects of the Incoming Soul and pregnant feet.

The Incoming Soul and Pregnant Feet

PRECONCEPTION

Incoming Soul (ICS)

Preconception for the Incoming Soul is a period when he conceive of and plans his human existence.
It is a time when he slows down his vibrations sufficiently to becom physical.

The mother

Some times people with clairvoyant vision can see this energy abo the mother. The author has not yet encountered anyone who can see the energy about the mother's feet. Please tell Susanne if someone has this experience.

CONCEPTION

Conception

Conception is the interface between spirit and matter.
In a split second the Incoming Soul retains his spirit and acquires the physical contributions from both mother and father. In that sing cell is the potential of an entire life. Truly awesome!

Physical

ICS is now a fertilised ovum, a single cell that carries the blueprint that not only give him his gender, his DNA, and genes, but also th tribal energies of both families.

Metaphysical aspect

At conception the lovingness or lack of loving, for example, rape h an effect on the mind, emotions and behaviour of the future perso

Pregnant feet

It is too early to observe this on the feet.

POST-CONCEPTION, DAYS 1 TO 7

Days 1 to 7

During days 1 to 7 rapid cell division takes place.
At the same time as the cells are dividing this group of cells (Moru is being carried along the fallopian tube.

Implantation

About seven days after conception the group of cells (now called a Blastocyst) implants in the lining of the uterus. Some women have physical sensation of implantation, but mostly it passes unnoticed.

Embryo

The Incoming Soul is now called an embryo. To maintain his physical presence (maintain the pregnancy) he makes the hormon - Human Chorionic Gonadotrophin (HCG).

The mother

One of the effects of HCG is that woman's periods stop. A week after implantation the woman misses her period and suspects that she is pregnant.

It is still too early to sense the pregnancy on the feet.

FIRST TRIMESTER OF PREGNANCY

WEEK 6

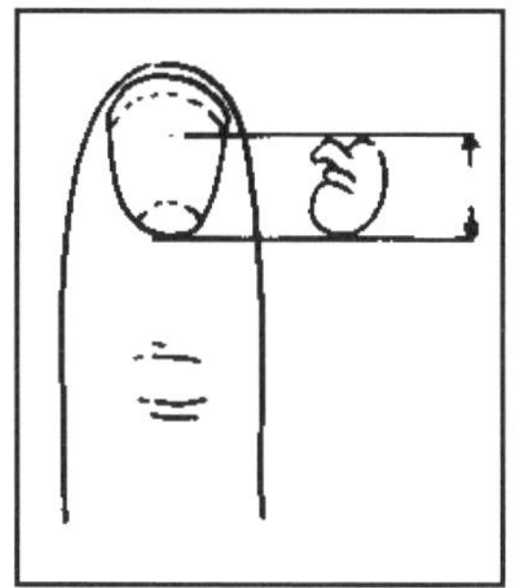

"At week 6 ICS is about 5 mm long from his head to his bottom, a bit smaller than his mum's little fingernail. His brain, stomach and intestines are developing and the heart is starting to beat. Little dimples on the head mark where the eyes and ears will be. Arms and legs are starting to bud". (NSW Health Department)

Metaphysical aspect

At this time while ICS is creating his body he is also establishing his metaphysical self.

He is totally aware of his mum's reactions: if she is thrilled to bits to have him or feels that it is the biggest mistake of her life and wants to be rid of him.

He is assembling his inner feelings and emotions - if all is well for him he will be calm and settled; if there are stresses he may have a great fear of the unknown.

Pregnant feet

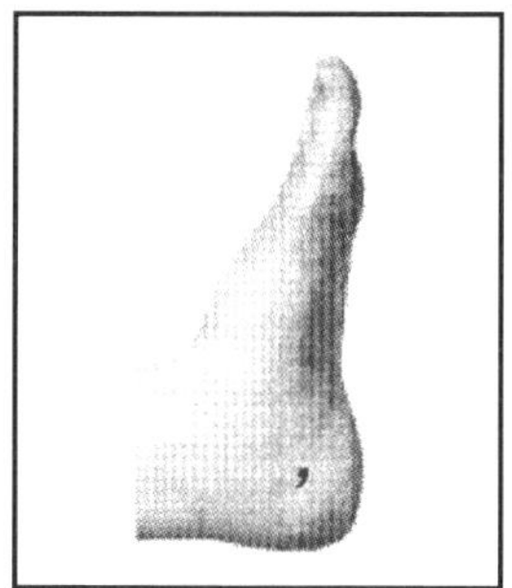

At about this time the pregnancy shows on the feet.
The earliest that the author has observed this phenomena is just after four weeks gestation.

The reflexion of the pregnancy on the feet looks like a comma that is a different colour from the background foot, for example, pink on a white foot or white on a dark foot.
It is located in the non-pregnant uterus reflex zone on one foot only. Some reflexologists feel that whichever foot the mark is on indicates the gender of the ICS - left foot female, right foot male. The author has observed that whichever foot the mark is on is the same side of the uterus that the ICS has implanted and so that is the site of the placenta.

After about six weeks the comma becomes a slight bulge. Some reflexologists can feel another energy in the uterus reflex zone, which they say is like warmth or coldness, a draft or more frequently a pulse.

WEEKS 8 AND 9

"At 8 to 9 weeks a face is forming, the eyes and ears are developing and embryo has a mouth and tongue. The heart, brain, lungs, kidneys, liver and intestines are all developing. Limbs are growing and hands show signs of fingers and feet show signs of toes." (NSW Health Department)

WEEK 10

The bones in the big toe ossify. At the same time so do the bones of the skull.
As reflexologists - wouldn't you just know it?

WEEK 12

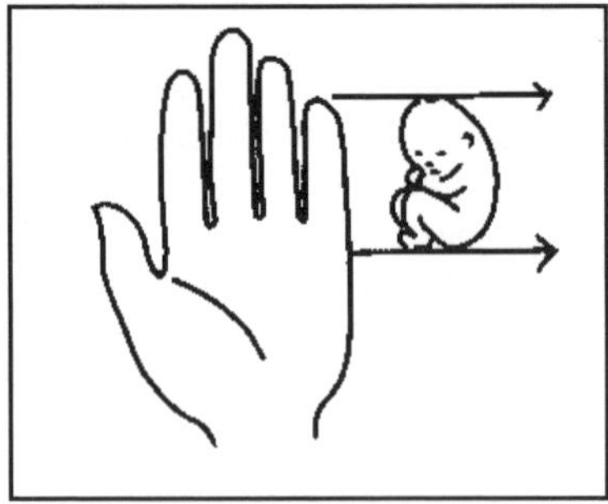

ICS *"is about 5 cm long from head to bottom i.e. about the size of a little finger"*. He has grown an entire body complete with nose and ovaries or testicles. (NSW Health Department)

He takes up nearly all of the space in the pelvis.

At the end of week 12 ICS has a name change; he is no longer an embryo and becomes a foetus.

Metaphysical aspect

ICS continues to merge his spiritual being with his physical life, the affects of which will last all his life.

Pregnant feet

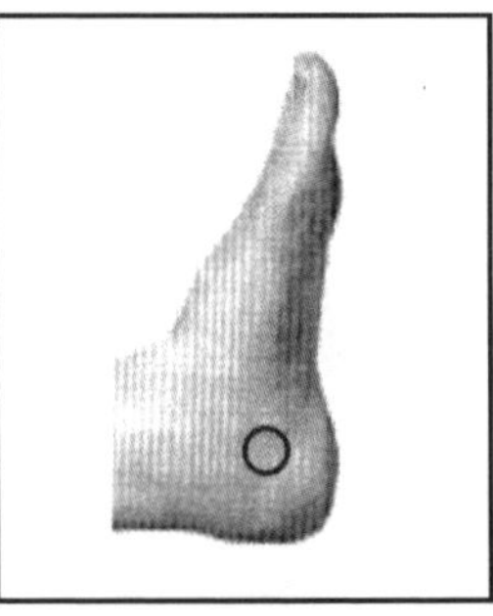

Over the past few weeks the comma has changed into a sphere and has enlarged. The growing sphere is palpable on the uterus reflex zone in the same position as the comma was.

SECOND TRIMESTER OF PREGNANCY

13 TO 14 WEEKS

The pelvis is no longer large enough to contain the growing pregnancy and the uterus with its contents move into the abdomen.

Author's experience

The author has palpated pregnant feet as the above movement was happening. The pregnant uterus reflex zone felt about the size of the end of a thumb and slid from under the palpating thumb into a position just above the groin line.

WEEK 16

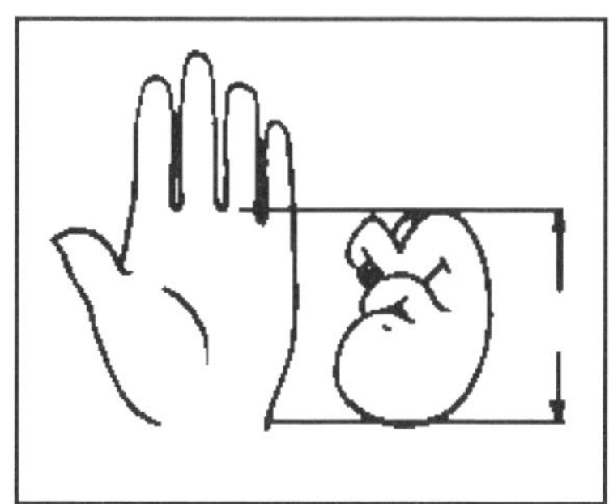

"At week 16 the foetus is about 10 cm long, from head to bottom - about the size of the palm of the hand." (NSW Health Department)

WEEK 16 TO 20

Quickening

At some time from 16 to 20 weeks the mother feels her baby move - quickening.

Incoming Soul

When the mother feels her baby move it marks a change for ICS. He has now completed the basics of his internal metaphysical foundation and begins to develop his outgoing nature.

Movement

He wriggles strongly enough for his mother to feel.
He sucks his thumb, gets hiccups, passes urine, swallows some amniotic fluid and if he is a boy even gets erections!

Sound

Living inside his mum is quite noisy for ICS; he hears his mum's heart beat, her breathing, talking, and her meal times i.e. her swallowing, digestion and things passing through her intestines. He is aware of sounds and eventually can differentiate between his parents, friends and music that he likes or dislikes. He reacts to loud noises.

Touch

As soon as ICS has hands and feet he can touch parts of his body. He learns to investigate things by touch. He frequently sucks his fingers or thumb.

Sensation

He responds to his mother's moods. He usually enjoys his mum having reflexology and lets her know if he does not like it. He responds to pain and anxiety.

Metaphysical aspect

This is a time of development. If all is well ICS will develop the idea of form and order. If there are stresses he may feel out of touch with the realities of life.

Pregnant feet

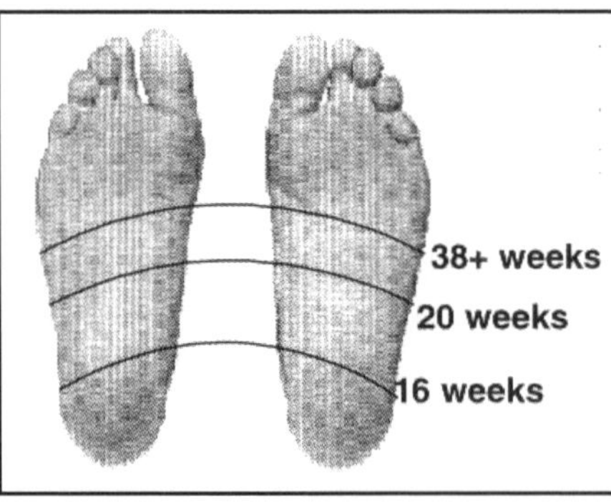

The pregnancy can be palpated on the abdominal reflex zones.

At 16 weeks it can be felt just above the groin line.

By 20 weeks it is at the level of the umbilicus reflex zone.

WEEK 24

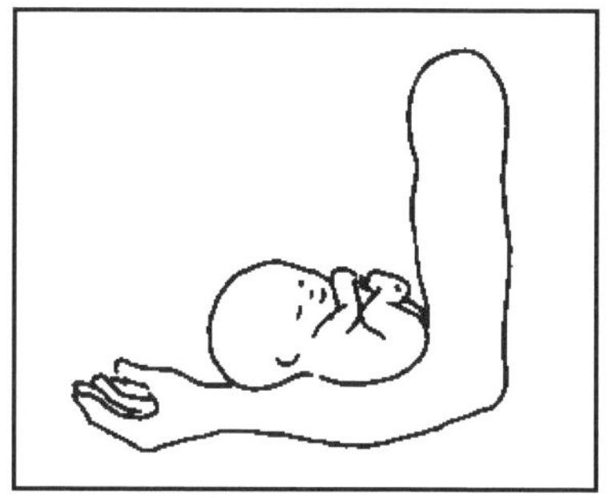

"At 24 weeks ICS is about 21 cm long from head to bottom, or about the length from the mother's wrist to her elbow". (NSW Health Department)

Pregnant feet

The pregnancy can be palpated on the abdominal reflex zones.

Many reflexologists can feel the "lie" of the baby on the feet. One foot feels as though it has more substantial energy - the solid part of the baby - his back.

The other foot may feel like action energy - the arms and legs.

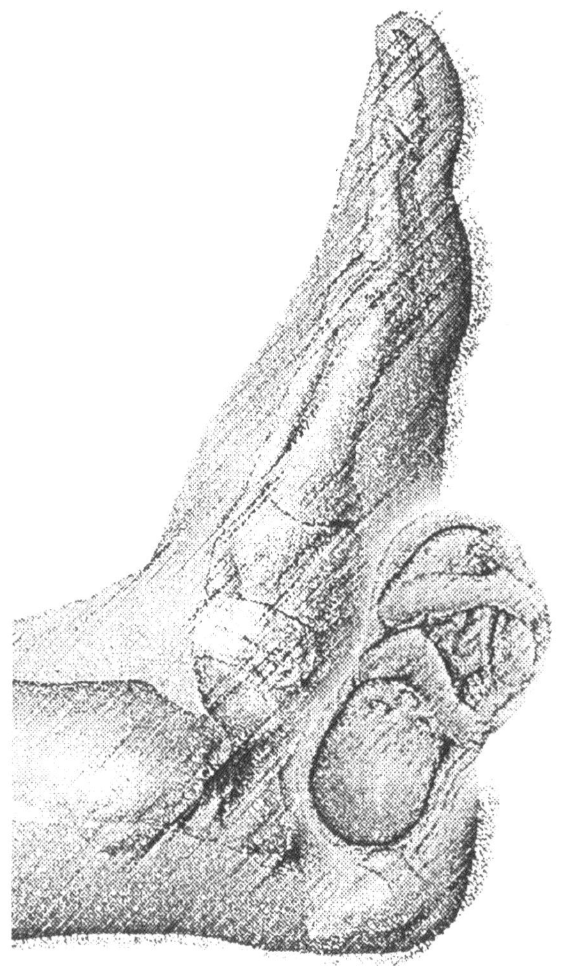

THIRD TRIMESTER OF PREGNANCY

WEEK 32

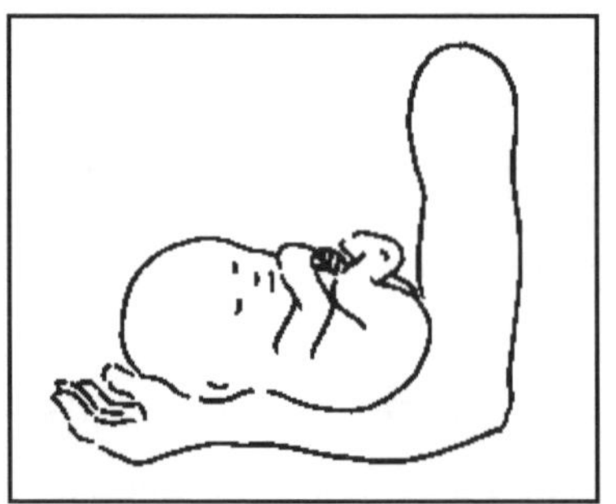

"At 32 weeks fetus (sic) is about 25 cm long from his head to his bottom, or about the length from the base of his mother's fingers to her elbow." (NSW Health Department)

Metaphysical aspect

ICS is now preparing for his birthing. If so far during his gestation all has gone well he will feel confident about his preparations. If there are stresses he may feel anxious about the next change and refuse to move forward.

Pregnant feet

Some reflexologists can tell the position of the baby - if he is head down or breech down.
Several reflexologists have said that they have a sense of baby movement and many reflexologists can sense the energy of the pregnancy several centimetres away from the sole and often it is possible to be aware of the vitality of the baby.

WEEK 40

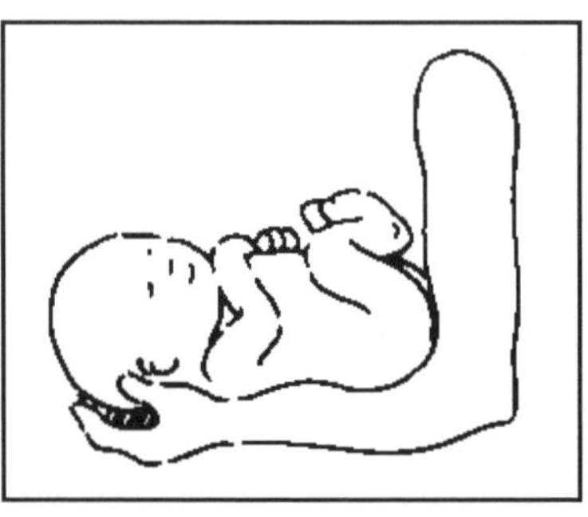

At 40 weeks ICS is due to be born and *"is about 33cm long from his head to his bottom, or about the length from the tips of his mother's fingers to her elbow".* (NSW Health Department)

Pregnant feet

The baby fills the abdomen and reflexologists sense that everything about the feet feels bounding full.

Some reflexologists can feel whether or not the baby's head is engaged.

Aren't reflexologists amazing!

BIRTHING

Physical experience

The Incoming Soul undergoes an impressive physical experience, he has to withstand huge pressures and squeeze through a passage that does not seem big enough.

The experience of birthing leaves a profound imprint on the person.

Recommended reading

The Metamorphic Technique was the topic at one of the seminars organised by the Association of Reflexologists (AoR) UK, Gaston Saint-Pierre spoke about the *"Types of Birth and the Way it Affects Us"*. The transcript is in Reflexions Journal of the Association of Reflexologists March 2003 Issue 70, page 2.

Pregnant feet

It is unlikely that the reflexologist will be able to observe the mother's feet at this time.

IMMEDIATE POSTNATAL

Within moments of birthing the Incoming Soul has to adapt to enormous changes. Some of these changes are:

Breathing

ICS leaves a fluid environment and has to swiftly adapt to an air environment and breathe.

Physically

The newborn must take in oxygen and excrete carbon dioxide through his lungs.

Metaphysically

With his first breath the individual is imprinted with his astrological natal chart.

Being severed

The umbilical cord is cut thus severing the newborn from his mother.

Physically

He is no longer dependent on his mother's blood supply and must instantly change his cardio-vascular system. Major circulatory changes take place.

Metaphysically

The life giving, enclosed dependence on his mother has ceased and he must live for himself.

Nourishment

He must now take in nourishment and have bowel movements.

Physically

The newborn must suck, swallow, digest, absorb and excrete for himself.

Metaphysically

His survival depends on his ability to adapt.

Warmth

In utero the temperature was fairly constant.

Physically

The newborn's heat-regulating system like many new things is inefficient.

Metaphysically

"It's cold out there" and it's easy for him to feel abandoned. He no longer has warmth and shelter.

POSTNATAL FEET

Reflexologist's experience

Reflexologists who have worked with clients in late pregnancy and again soon after birthing are always amazed at the enormous instant change in the feet.

Reflexology Techniques

INFORMATION GATHERING ABOUT PREGNANT FEET

Over the years many reflexologists have observed the energy of the pregnancy in the feet. Some reflexologists have developed an amazing sensing of those energies. Some of these methods to gather information about pregnant feet are given below.

SENSING

To gain a general impression of the pregnancy:

Method

Use the tips of all the fingers or the "solar plexus" of both hands. Lightly touching, stroke over the reflex zones for the internal pelvis, along the spine and across the abdomen. At first it may take a while to sense any energy. It is easier not to look. Once you can sense energy allow your fingers or hands to move freely, stopping where they will to give you information. It is not necessary to have a logical interpretation of what you are sensing; a felt sense or intuition will give you a more profound understanding.

PALPATING

Palpating can be used to feel the fundal height, the lie and position of the baby.

Method

To palpate the fundal height (the level of the top of the uterus): hold both feet with your thumbs across the groin line and fingers resting on the dorsal aspect of the feet. Move the thumbs up the abdominal reflex zones towards the diaphragm reflex zones. Use the length of the thumbs to feel where there is a change of tissue tone. That change gives you an idea about the fundal height.

To palpate the lie of the baby: use the tips of your fingers to feel on which foot the abdominal reflex zone feels more solid and which feels less solid. The side that feels more solid is the side where the baby has his back.

To palpate the position of the baby: use your fingertips to feel a firm circular area about the size of the end of your thumb. This will give information about where the baby's head is and if he is head up or head down. This last palpation is not easy.

IMAGING

Sometimes it is possible to "see" the pregnancy. Look at the soles of the feet with an unfocused gaze; some reflexologists can "see" the baby and get an impression of his well being.
If the mother has fairly pink soles use a "windscreen wiper" type movement across the abdominal reflex zones - you may get a "picture" of the baby.

These are a few ways the author uses to gather information about pregnant feet.
The reflexologist is encouraged to discover more ways. Remember we are only limited by our imaginations!

Part 5: Birthing

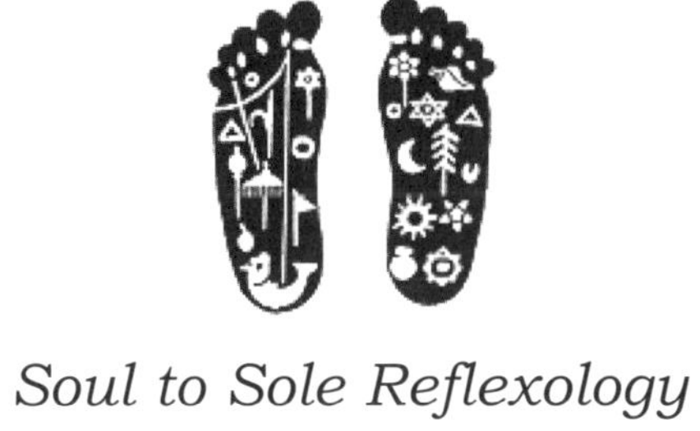

Soul to Sole Reflexology

YOUR CLIENT

As this is about you the reflexologist preparing to be a support person during birthing, you need to be prepared for how long the job will take.

Expected Date of Delivery (EDD)

Your client may go into labour any time from two weeks before her EDD to two weeks after.
This means that you will need to set aside four weeks to be on call and ready to attend. During that time your client needs to be able to contact you at any time of the day or night. Therefore she needs your mobile phone number or know where you are and how she can contact you.

Your preparation:

- Be available; do not book a holiday during that period
- Be fit; do not get squiffy at a party.

Where

Where are you going to work with your client?

- Will you work with your client at her home?
- Will you go with her to the hospital?

Caution

Do not take your client to hospital in your car. Your professional reflexology insurance will not cover you to transport her.
As a friend you may take her but as a client you must not.

Length of labour

How long is a labour?
There is no way you can tell.

Questions to consider:

- Will you stay throughout - however long it takes?
- Will you stay overnight?
- Will you work 9am to 5pm?

Make arrangements

You need to make arrangements for:

- Your family: meals, school collecting, husband, pets etc.
- Your work.
- Your social life.

All the arrangements will need to be able to be activated at a moment's notice.

Promises

Never make promises to your client that you cannot keep. Always be up-front with what you can and cannot do, for example, in the birthing room the reflexologist must **never** make birthing procedure decisions.
A frequently encountered problem is if you promise to "not let them give her an epidural", however an epidural later becomes necessary.

REST OF THE TEAM

The rest of the team are other people who are important to your client.

Partner

It is better to have met your client's partner before she begins birthing.
Birthing can be very traumatic for the partner. He sees his best most loved person in all the world going through the most incredible experience. He may feel out of his depth, inadequate, keen to help but not know what to do and is powerless to influence anything. Once your client is under way, biology takes over. But be prepared for your client's partner reaction - he does not have Mother Nature on his side and may need more of your attention than your client.

Children

Occasionally children are at a hospital birth, you are more likely to encounter them at a home birth. Children need special consideration, as they're young lives are about to change forever. Frequently they are the least worried people.
If the children are to be present at the birth is part of your job to look after them?

Parents

The clients mother is the person to empathise with, she will probably have an emotional explosion.

Professionals

The obstetric team are totally in charge of the health and well being of both mother and baby.

Write

Write to the professionals to inform them of your client's wish for you to be her support person.

Write to:

- The obstetrician Address him/her by his/her full title (include name and qualifications).
- The Nursing Unit Manager of the Maternity Division.
- The Midwifery Unit Manager of the Birthing Unit.
- Independent Midwife (if your client is having a home birth).

Include in the letter

In the letter include:

- Your client's name and address, her EDD.
- Your name and address.
- A photocopy of your reflexology qualifications.
- A photocopy of your insurance (you are not covered by the hospital insurance).
- Health benefits provider number (for Australian refelxologists).

Advantage

The great advantage of writing to the professionals is that not only is it courteous but also when you arrive at the birthing room the staff will be expecting you and know your name.

The midwife

For working with the midwife see page 126.

Introduction to Birthing

Birthing is a momentous time. It is a time of great highs and lows. Both mother and baby will end a very close encounter with each other, go through an enormous experience and begin a life that is new to both of them.

Birthing care

Midwives undertake birthing care. It is highly specialised skilled work.

The mother

The mother's body under the influence of the hormones of pregnancy will have prepared itself. Her other antenatal preparation will have given her some knowledge and confidence in her birthing skills. If she has been having reflexology she will be in the best condition possible for whatever type of birthing she will undergo.
Her emotions can range from thrill and excitement to absolute terror.
For the first time mother this time of transition from Maid to Mother is like an initiation and is a life changing experience.
For subsequent birthings it is still a momentous occasion.

The Incoming Soul

The Incoming Soul has completed his physical growth and is mature. He is also metaphysically prepared. Some babies can't wait to get out while others are reluctant to move.
How he carries out the action of his birthing will imprint on his psyche it will affect how he carries out actions for the rest of his life. For example he may be born purposefully and steadily, or be reluctant to put in an appearance or arrive with gusto.
Passing through the birth canal may cause him fear and anxiety or he may have the confidence to know he can handle it. Physically and emotionally he may suffer trauma or be able to let the birthing power help him.

The father

Nowadays there are many expectations put on the father. He is expected to be present at the birth, be supportive and understanding in an environment that is alien to him. He has to cope with a mass of emotional conflicts.

Reflexology

Naturally reflexology has a place in a birthing room. Many midwives use reflexology as one of their skills.
For reflexologists planning to be a birthing support person in addition to their reflexology skills there are several extra things to bear in mind, which will be considered in this module.

Wise words from the author

"I feel that a few words of wisdom are needed here; we (reflexologists) cannot know the greater power that directs life. There are occasions during birthing that even with the best preparation appear to be terrible. There are many things that affect the birthing process and the outcome that cannot be predicted such as the response of the client's personality and attitude under stress and her belief systems e.g. that her mother and grand mother have had long hard labours and she will be the same. Her Karma or some spiritual testing may affect her.
My wisdom for the reflexologist is - know that you have contributed your love, care, knowledge and skills and accept that there are things over which you have no control."

Preparation

REFLEXOLOGIST'S PREPARATION TO BE A BIRTHING SUPPORT PERSON

As part of their care some reflexologists like to attend their client's birthing as a support person. This work is fantastic, amazing, breathtaking, emotional, poignant, exhausting, and rewarding, however it is essential that the reflexologist is well prepared as being a support person is like negotiating a minefield.

The following are some known dilemmas that need to be addressed and some suggestions to help.

YOU THE REFLEXOLOGIST

Ideally you need to be centred, grounded, calm, knowledgeable, skilled and caring!

When working with such a miraculous process such as birthing expect to experience the full range of feelings and emotions. If you have buttons to press they will be pressed. So first consider yourself.

Personal stuff

Why do you want to be present?

Skills

Be clear what skills you are prepared to use, such as reflexology, husband / child support, tea making and so on. Set boundaries or you will be asked to do all sorts of things.

Strengths

Be very clear about your strengths. You will need to call on them for yourself, your client and her family.

Vulnerabilities

Here is where your buttons will be pressed. It is helpful to know in advance and take self-care action.

Needs

Remember you too have needs. Consider what will you do about food, sleep and toilet needs.
Food, will you take a picnic, go to the canteen - if so where is it and does it have closing times or will you go home for meals?
Rest / Sleep, will you doze in the room, go home for the night or miss out altogether?
Toilet needs, where is the nearest public loo? Does it close at night?

Recognition

It is so important that for the skilled, loving work that you are to do there is a form of recognition of you. It does not matter what form it takes as long as it is meaningful to you.

Fees - if you require a fee it must be negotiated well beforehand (it is not a good time once your client is in labour).

Some options for negotiating a fee are:

- A set hourly rate. This is not always satisfactory, as no one knows how many hours it will take and it may become too expensive.
- A set fee for the entire session. The problem here is that you may be over or under paid.

Gift - you may choose to accept a gift - your client needs to know that is acceptable to you.

Complimentary - you may choose to attend the birth and that in itself is your reward.

YOUR CLIENT

As this is about you the reflexologist preparing to be a support person during birthing, you need to be prepared for how long the job will take.

Expected Date of Delivery (EDD)

Your client may go into labour any time from two weeks before her EDD to two weeks after.
This means that you will need to set aside four weeks to be on call and ready to attend. During that time your client needs to be able to contact you at any time of the day or night. Therefore she needs your mobile phone number or know where you are and how she can contact you.

Your preparation:

- Be available; do not book a holiday during that period
- Be fit; do not get squiffy at a party.

Where

Where are you going to work with your client?

- Will you work with your client at her home?
- Will you go with her to the hospital?

Caution

Do not take your client to hospital in your car. Your professional reflexology insurance will not cover you to transport her.
As a friend you may take her but as a client you must not.

Length of labour

How long is a labour?
There is no way you can tell.

Questions to consider:

- Will you stay throughout - however long it takes?
- Will you stay overnight?
- Will you work 9am to 5pm?

Make arrangements

You need to make arrangements for:

- Your family: meals, school collecting, husband, pets etc.
- Your work.
- Your social life.

All the arrangements will need to be able to be activated at a moment's notice.

Promises

Never make promises to your client that you cannot keep. Always be up-front with what you can and cannot do, for example, in the birthing room the reflexologist must **never** make birthing procedure decisions.
A frequently encountered problem is if you promise to "not let them give her an epidural", however an epidural later becomes necessary.

REST OF THE TEAM

The rest of the team are other people who are important to your client.

Partner

It is better to have met your client's partner before she begins birthing.
Birthing can be very traumatic for the partner. He sees his best most loved person in all the world going through the most incredible experience. He may feel out of his depth, inadequate, keen to help but not know what to do and is powerless to influence anything.
Once your client is under way, biology takes over. But be prepared for your client's partner reaction - he does not have Mother Nature on his side and may need more of your attention than your client.

Children

Occasionally children are at a hospital birth, you are more likely to encounter them at a home birth. Children need special consideration, as they're young lives are about to change forever. Frequently they are the least worried people.
If the children are to be present at the birth is part of your job to look after them?

Parents

The clients mother is the person to empathise with, she will probably have an emotional explosion.

Professionals

The obstetric team are totally in charge of the health and well being of both mother and baby.

Write

Write to the professionals to inform them of your client's wish for you to be her support person.

Write to:

- The obstetrician Address him/her by his/her full title (include name and qualifications).
- The Nursing Unit Manager of the Maternity Division.
- The Midwifery Unit Manager of the Birthing Unit.
- Independent Midwife (if your client is having a home birth).

Include in the letter

In the letter include:

- Your client's name and address, her EDD.
- Your name and address.
- A photocopy of your reflexology qualifications.
- A photocopy of your insurance (you are not covered by the hospital insurance).
- Health benefits provider number (for Australian refelxologists).

Advantage

The great advantage of writing to the professionals is that not only is it courteous but also when you arrive at the birthing room the staff will be expecting you and know your name.

The midwife

For working with the midwife see page 126.

OTHER PRACTICAL STUFF

Car park

Check that you know:

- Where it is.
- Is there a charge - if so be sure you have the money available.
- Does it close at night.

Security

The hospital may be locked at night - if so:

- How will you get in?
- Do you need a pass?

Insurance

The hospital insurance only covers its own staff. It does not cover visiting specialists.
Ensure you have insurance to cover you.

So you are going to do a job that you do not know when it will begin or how long it will take, you will be in a different environment from usual and you do not know with whom you will be working!

Birthing

THE BIG DAY

Early in pregnancy women are given a date for when they will probably birth their baby. It is known as EDD (expected date of delivery). However it is quite unusual for the woman to have her baby on that day. Most women go into labour within ten days before or after that date.

It is thought that the Incoming Soul sets the start of birthing with an intricate interaction of hormones.

Prodromal signs of birthing	Some of the prodromal signs of approaching birthing: ● The baby moves down the birth canal and becomes less active. ● The mother becomes more active and has nesting instincts. ● The Braxton Hicks contractions become regular and stronger. ● The mother has diarrhoea.
Note	It is very rare for a woman to go into labour without any warning.
False labour	There may be several false starts to birthing.
Reflexology	If possible give full reflexology sessions to keep her relaxed and grounded. Remember having had reflexology your client will be in the best condition for whatever kind of birthing she has.
Note	Although reflexology will help your client be in the best condition for whatever kind of birthing she has, remember that you cannot guarantee a painless, easy birthing.
Imminent signs birthing commencing	The mother has a "show"; she passes some blood and mucus from her vagina. The contractions are regular. With a vaginal examination the midwives can tell that the cervix is opening.

STAGES OF LABOUR

First stage of labour

The first stage of labour is from when the contractions are regular and the cervix is dilating, until the cervix is fully dilated.

Second stage of labour

The second stage of labour is the expulsion of the baby.

Third stage of labour

The third stage of labour is the delivery of the placenta.

FIRST STAGE OF LABOUR

THE LATENT PHASE

The latent phase or early labour can take several hours.

The client

The client is often excited and apprehensive. Her contractions although regular may be more than five minutes apart and are bearable.

Reflexology

This may be the longest reflexology session ever! Pace yourself.
It is easy to be carried away with the thrill of it all but remember it may be several hours duration.
If possible be with the client at her home. Be very adaptable with the reflexology - do a little whenever it seems a good time.
An ideal situation is to do a relaxing twenty minutes or so and the client sleeps for the rest of the latent phase.

Better condition

The client will be in better condition if she is well rested and can stay out of hospital for as long as possible.

How to know when to go to hospital

Go to hospital if the client:

- Is bleeding from her vagina.
- Has a rupture of membranes (waters break).
- Is worried / anxious and would feel safer there.
- Can't talk through a contraction.

Any queries

If you have any queries or worries phone who ever will be in charge of the birthing: the hospital birthing suite, team midwives or independent midwife.

ESTABLISHED LABOUR

Established labour is when the contractions are probably less than five minutes apart and the cervix is probably more than five centimetres dilated. The word 'probably' is used, as there are no exact parameters for measuring established labour, as it is an individual event.

Management of labour

The management of labour varies with each client and is dependent on:

- The health and well being of mother and baby.
- The midwife's skill.
- Hospital policy.
- Wishes of the client.

WORKING WITH THE MIDWIFE

The responsibility of the midwife / obstetrician is total intrapartum care that is the health and wellbeing of both mother and baby.

Midwife in charge

The midwife is totally in charge of the case and the reflexologist must work under her direction.
Usually the midwife is welcoming to a support person especially when he/she sees the benefits of reflexology.

Make birthing decisions

The reflexologist must never make birthing procedure decisions.
There will be obstetric procedures that the reflexologist may not comprehend and is not entitled to an explanation.
There may be occasions when the reflexologist is requested to discontinue treatment or leave the room.

Inform midwife

The reflexologist must always keep the midwife informed of what they are doing.
A simple explanation of reflexology will usually suffice.
Good communication with the midwife is beneficial to all.

Never dose

The reflexologist must never dose the client with anything e.g. homeopathic or Bach flower remedies unless agreed to by the midwife.

WORKING WITH THE CLIENT

The overall aim of birthing care is to work with natural rhythms instead of trying to control, suppress or alter them. Birthing has a strong natural rhythm.

Great advantage

The great advantage for the client is that she already knows her support person and the benefits of reflexology.

Relax

Keep the client relaxed so that nature can take its course.
Use any relaxation techniques.

Fear

Fear is one of the feelings that can stop a labour. Fear can be caused by the birthing itself, or by something like someone entering the room.
Use "Solar plexus" hold and sedate the adrenal glands reflex zones and more relaxation techniques.

Keep prowling

It is better for the client if she keeps upright and prowling about.
One of the subtle energies of the feet is that the Mother Principle is located in the heels. (Metamorphic Technique, Gaston Saint Pierre).
When a woman is birthing she is doing her ultimate mothering endeavour. To gain benefit from this knowledge ensure your client keeps her heels on the ground, then her Mother Principle is gaining energy from Mother Earth.
There is however a small problem for the reflexologist - he/she cannot get to the feet! Now is a perfect time for Vertical Reflexology Technique (VRT). See recommended reading, page 188.

Don't touch

During birthing some women attain a state similar to bliss and are totally inwardly attuned. They have so much internal sensory stimulation and need total external sensory deprivation, that is no noise (music), no aromas, no touching and keep eyes closed.
It also includes no reflexology! This is one of those occasions when the system is working successfully - don't fix it! Be prepared for masterly inactivity.

Toes pull back

Towards the end of the first stage of labour the woman's toes pull back (go into extreme dorsiflexion). When she is ready to push her toes go into extreme plantarflexion.
From the foot reading point of view it is as though the client is pulling back from a situation then rushing forward into another.

TRANSITION

Transition is an in-between time. It is the end of the first stage of labour and the second stage has not yet begun. The woman emerges from her inward looking state and gathers energy to birth her baby.

Reflexology

It is unlikely that the practitioner can do any reflexology at this time.

Warning

Women often become tempestuous during transition and may swear, scratch and bite. Keep out of the way and accept it as part of the experience. It is not a personal insult to you and your client will not remember it.

SECOND STAGE OF LABOUR

The second stage of labour is from when the cervix is fully dilated until the baby is born.

The woman	Some women find this stage terrifying with the feeling of being overtaken by unseen forces. Other women revel in the thrill of it all and love the experience and feel more in control with the intense urge to push.
The midwife	This is yet another time for of the midwife to use her skill.
The reflexologist	It is unlikely that the reflexologist can "do" reflexology. However the support person can brandish the cooling cloths! And keep an eye on the partner. It is probably best to keep out of the way.

THE NEWBORN

The miracle	The reflexologist will probably burst into tears! He/she has been witnessing a miracle and feels swamped by the wonder of it all.
Observe	Almost before the mother does any thing else she looks at and fondles her baby's feet!

THIRD STAGE OF LABOUR

The third stage of labour is the delivery of the placenta.

The woman	The third stage of labour is lovely. The woman has her baby in her arms and hardly notices the placenta slip out.
The midwife	This is more skilled midwife work.
The reflexologist	Keep admiring the baby.

RETAINED PLACENTA

Occasionally the placenta does not become severed from the wall of the uterus and cannot be delivered - a retained placenta.

Obstetric care	If the placenta still does not separate after the midwife has tried several manoeuvres, the treatment is for the woman to have it manually removed under a general anaesthetic.
Reflexologist	The reflexologist can inform the midwife that there is a reflexology technique that may help.
Reflexology	Bi-manually strongly stimulate the non-pregnant uterus reflex zones. Bi-manually strongly stimulate the hypothalamus reflex zones.

POST TERM

The Incoming Soul is thought to create the onset of labour. Usually women go into labour spontaneously at a time within two weeks either side of their EDD. Some pregnancies continue beyond the EDD.

GENERAL INFORMATION

Post-term

The term used when a woman has passed her EDD is post-term.

Reasons for a prolonged pregnancy

There are reasons for a prolonged pregnancy - the dates may be wrong or the woman may have a long menstrual cycle.
The baby may not be ready.

Associated risks

There are risks associated with post term pregnancy:

- The placenta is designed to work efficiently for forty weeks, after that time it starts to decline.
- The baby's well being is compromised.

Closely monitor

The obstetric team will closely monitor progress.
If there are no problems the pregnancy continues until the woman naturally goes into labour.

Induction of labour

If there are problems the obstetrician will decide to do an induction of labour.

Women's experience

A high percentage of women who have experienced induction of labour would not like the experience repeated.

SOME NATURAL METHODS TO HELP BIRTHING BEGIN

Remember there is no method that guarantees success.

The well-known methods

Suggest that the client has "a hot curry, a hot motor bike ride and hot sex"! Not necessarily all of them or in that order!

Guided visualisation

Many reflexologists are multi-skilled and include in their expertise guided visualisation. Reflexologists who use that skill will find it particularly useful to use with a client who has gone post-term.

Note

Guided visualisation is helpful throughout pregnancy and especially during the preparation for birthing.

Reflexology Techniques

REFLEXOLOGY PRIMING LABOUR

Reflexology priming labour is strongly stimulating specific reflexology reflex zones with the intention of creating a boost of energy to encourage the onset of labour contractions.

Caution

PRIMING LABOUR IS NOT A DECISION TO BE MADE BY THE REFLEXOLOGY THERAPIST

CRITERIA FOR USE

Essential

THE CLIENT MUST BE POST-TERM.

Consultation

It is important to have full consultation with the client and her obstetric caregivers.
If there are any obstetric problems obtain the obstetric caregiver's written permission

Note

Denise Tiran a Reflex Zone Therapist and the Principal Lecturer in Complementary Medicine / Midwifery, School of Health at the University of Greenwich, UK, has developed the skill of predicting the imminence of labour using the reflex zones of the feet.

Recommended reading

Clinical Reflexology, a Guide for Health Professionals by Peter Mackereth & Denise Tiran

Many women who are post-term and have no problems respond well to the reflexology priming of labour.

PROCEDURE

BEGIN THE SESSION

Reflexology

Relaxation techniques	Use lots of relaxation techniques - to relax body and mind to accept that the inevitable will happen.
Endocrine balance	To prepare the endocrine system for its vital role to prime labour.
Listen	Listen to the client - she may express fears and doubts that are preventing her from the onset of labour.
Positive language	Always use positive language to encourage the client's confidence in her birthing ability.

PRIMING TECHNIQUES

Work the primary techniques for about fifteen minutes.

Reflexology	
Hypothalamus reflex zone	Use hook and back-up technique - for stimulation, integration and response from the brain's brain.
Pituitary reflex zone	Stimulate strongly - to set the body messengers working.
Large intestine especially rectum reflex zones	Stimulate strongly - to encourage pelvic outflow action (this mimics the effects of the old fashioned enema).
Internal pelvic reflex zones	Stimulate strongly - to work up some action.
Hips and pelvis reflex zones	Vigorous ankle boogie - to shake things up.
Acupressure points*	For location see Part 3, Pregnancy page 49. Stimulate Spleen 6 and Bladder 60 - to expedite labour. Stimulate Bladder 67 - to give the baby energy.
Note	*These points are not reflex zones they are part of Traditional Chinese Medicine (TCM). Their use is recommended as they are effective and fall within the foot reflex zones area.

END THE SESSION

Reflexology	
Relaxation techniques	Use lots of relaxation techniques - to relax body and mind to accept that the inevitable will happen.
Endocrine balance	To prepare it for its vital role.

EXPECTED OUTCOME

No guarantee

There is no guarantee that the body will respond. However even with a medical induction of labour there is no guarantee of success.

The author

The author has found that clients begin contracting in about an hour after the session. Most of them carry on into established labour. For some a repeat session is required.

Midwives

Midwives who use this technique have found that after the technique is used in the antenatal clinic, the clients go home and fall asleep! They wake several hours later in established labour.

Introduction to Postnatal Care

The agony and ecstasy of birthing can leave a woman feeling jubilant, exhausted, sore and sick, full of disbelief and wonder and many other conflicting and confusing emotions and feelings.

The balancing, harmonising, and restoring qualities of reflexology therapy are superb at this time. Even if a woman has had a straightforward, uneventful birthing, her entire system will appreciate being balanced back to a non-pregnant state, and after all that hard work she deserves a reflexology session! If a woman has had a hard labour or traumatic experience the qualities of reflexology therapy will help enormously.

Author's opinion

Yes I know that you have read it before BUT in the opinion of the author reflexology and its practitioners are second to none for postnatal care.

What Elsa says

Gentle words of wisdom from the co-author of *Maternity Reflexology a Guide for Reflexologists*, by Elsa Reid and Susanne Enzer. Reproduced here with Elsa's blessings.

Natural therapy

Reflexology, a natural therapy, naturally supports the client's body, mind and spirit returning to a non-pregnant state.

Reflexologist

Immediate postnatal care is thrilling for the reflexologist. He/she gets to hear the Birthing Story as no one else will hear it.
It is great to complete a nine-month session!
It is delightful to know that whatever he/she did was an important piece in the events for an Incoming Soul.

The Postnatal Period

The postnatal period (puerperium) is the time from the end of birthing until six to eight weeks later when the woman's reproductive organs have returned to a non-pregnant state.

It is a time of yet more huge changes in body, mind and spirit.

THE FIRST POSTNATAL REFLEXOLOGY SESSION

The optimum time

The first or third days after birthing are the optimum time for the first postnatal reflexology session.

Time for reflexology

It is not always easy for a new mum to have time for reflexology. There are so many demands on her time: the baby, her husband, visitors, midwives, hospital routine, and so on.

Pick a time

Endeavour to choose a time when there are no other distractions.

Birthing Story

It is a great sadness to the author that so many times the new mum who has been through the most colossal experience of her life - especially first time mums - has no one to listen to her Birthing Story. Dear Maternity Reflexologists please listen to it.
Bring the flowers, admire the baby but most importantly LISTEN.

Reflexology

If possible give a full reflexology session and include:

- Lots of relaxation techniques - to help her readjust.
- Reflexology endocrine balance - to balance her return to a non-pregnant state.
- Reflexology lymphatic technique - to encourage the body to remove the remnants of pregnancy.
- "Solar plexus" hold - to vitalise and empower.

Reflexology Postnatal Care

GENERAL WELLBEING

Reflexology sessions

In an ideal situation a reflexology session each week is an excellent way to help the mother "get back on her feet". However this is not often attainable, new mothers have very little time to themselves. Consider shorter sessions.

Client comfort

The reflexologist needs to be adaptable to ensure his/her client comfort. Sometimes the client cannot sit - be prepared for VRT or have the client in a prone position.
The client may need to change her position frequently - be prepared for fidgets.

The baby

The client may choose to have her baby lying on her during the session. Usually both mother and baby sleep peacefully - ensure the baby does not roll off.

Reflexology

In each session include:

- Lots of relaxation techniques - to help her readjust.
- Reflexology endocrine balance - to balance her return to a non-pregnant state.
- Reflexology lymphatic technique - to encourage the body to remove the remnants of pregnancy.
- "Solar plexus" hold - to vitalise and empower.
- Reflexology therapy for specific conditions (if appropriate).

Postnatal Reflexology Therapy

AFTER DIFFERENT TYPES OF BIRTHING

NORMAL VAGINAL DELIVERY

Normal vaginal delivery is a birthing where the baby birthed head first with his chin tucked in, through the birth canal (vagina) without instrumental assistance and arrived in good condition.

Reflexology	
Entire body	All relaxations - to ease muscle fatigue and reduce tension.
Endocrine system	Endocrine balance - to create balance now that placental hormone production has ceased.
Lymphatic system	Lymphatic technique - to assist the body's removal of extra wastes.
Urinary system	"Flush" - to support the body's removal of extra fluid.

Also see "The first postnatal reflexology session"

AFTER INDUCTION OF LABOUR

An induction of labour is the medical method of making a woman go into labour. There are several methods that can be used depending on the woman's readiness to start labour.

After induction of labour many women feel that by the time labour commenced they were not in a good state and that the speed of events left them feeling out of control.

Reflexology	
Entire body	All relaxations - to ease the stresses.
"Solar plexus"	Calming hold - to restore her own life force.
Balance organ & "sense of self"	Link - to restore her "sense of self".
Liver	Stimulate - to aid removal of toxins.

AFTER FORCEPS DELIVERY OR VACUUM EXTRACTION

Forceps delivery and vacuum extraction are instrumental deliveries that are performed by the obstetrician.

Forceps

Forceps are used to assist the descent and / or rotation of the baby through the birth canal during the second stage of labour.

The mother

The mother will feel bruised and sore, especially if an episiotomy has been performed.

The baby

The baby may have facial bruising from the forceps and possibly trauma caused by a prolonged second stage of labour or foetal distress which may have necessitated the use of forceps.
The baby may have bruising and oedema on the part of his head from the vacuum attachment.

Reflexology

Internal pelvis	Healing hold - to promote healing. Linking hips, "solar plexus" and hypothalamus - to balance energy.
Sacral curve	Trigger point release - to ease the pain and clear blocked energies.
Perineum	Sedate - to promote healing.
"Solar plexus"	Bimanual hold - to restore calm.

What Elsa says

"Help the client come to terms with the reason for the use of forceps. Give TLC +++ if she is separated from her baby due to admission to the special / intensive care baby nursery".

Also see

After traumatic delivery, page 158.

AFTER MULTIPLE BIRTH

A multiple birth is twins or more. Frequently they are pre-term births. Many are vaginal deliveries and some are Caesarean section (C/S).

Reflexology

Uterus	Stimulate - to encourage involution.
Lymphatic system	Lymphatic technique - to reduce oedema and make the client feel good.
Spine	Massage and spinal twist - to relieve tension.
Pelvic floor and perineum	Stimulate - to strengthen.

Note

If the client has had forceps delivery, epidural anaesthesia, Caesarean section, include reflexology therapy for those situations in the treatment.

AFTER PRECIPITATE DELIVERY

A precipitate delivery is one that happens very quickly. It usually takes the mother unawares.

Reflexology	
Uterus	Stimulate - to encourage contractility.
Balance organ & "sense of self"	Link - to balance a being who feels out of "sync" with herself.
Endocrine system	Endocrine balance - to balance the hormones.
Spine	Spine runs (down) - to ground her.

AFTER PROLONGED LABOUR

Prolonged labour is one that may have taken more than twenty-four hours and in some instances several days.

Reflexology	
Entire body	Relaxations - to relieve tension and encourage rest.
Uterus	Stimulate - to increase contractility.
Chest	Dolphin - to help her "go with the flow".
Diaphragm	Pivot along - to release tension and emotions and to give her time to "debrief".
Note	Add spine runs (up) if she requires energising rather than relaxation e.g. to feed baby or visit baby in SCBU.

Also see Exhaustion, fatigue, page 155.

After a difficult or traumatic delivery, an unexpected outcome of an emotionally traumatic delivery, see Psychological aspects, page 158.`

AFTER LOWER SEGMENT CAESAREAN SECTION (C/S)

Lower segment Caesarean section (C/S) is the surgical delivery of the baby through the abdomen of the mother.

Reasons	C/S deliveries are necessary for a number of reasons. They may be planned because of a non-urgent problem, or unplanned arising from an emergency situation.
1. Mother	The mother's pelvic cavity is smaller than the baby's head.
2. Baby	The baby is too stressed to safely tolerate labour and / or vaginal delivery.
Anaesthetic	Except in emergency situations, most mothers are given the option of a general anaesthetic (GA) or an epidural anaesthetic.
Incision	The majority of C/S incisions are made horizontally (bikini line) and healing is excellent.
Out of bed	Even with a "drip", urinary catheter or wound drain, women are encouraged to get out of bed the same day as the C/S to reduce the risk of DVT.
"Wind"	Abdominal wind pain can be very uncomfortable.
Recommended	For at least six weeks after C/S it is recommended that the mother does not strain, lift, carry heavy weights or drive a car.
The parents	Parents may easily adjust to the idea of a C/S or may grieve for the normal vaginal delivery, which they could not have.

Reflexology

Non pregnant uterus	Healing hold - to allow healing energy to flow.
"Solar plexus"	Hold - to calm and centre.
Spine	Gentle spinal twist - to loosen stiffness.
Lungs / chest	Fish, dolphin, metatarsal stretches, lung press - to re-establish healthy breathing patterns.
Large intestines	Wind screen wipers - to help move "wind".
Splenic flexure	Massage - a really good spot to move "wind".
Lymphatic system	Lymphatic technique - to promote the removal of toxins.
Endocrine system	Balance - to restore balance as soon as possible.

Also see	After general anaesthetic - respiratory system.
What Elsa says	*"Be understanding about the client's reduced ability to move and encourage early mobilisation. Offer practical suggestions to reduce muscle strain e.g. bath the baby in the sink! Home visits could be a great idea."*

Body Systems

Women have wonderful powers of recovery. Throughout pregnancy and birthing there have been huge changes, now the woman's body, mind and spirit restores itself to its non-pregnant state and prepares for possible future babies!

The following information is arranged in body systems.

Each system includes	Postnatal physiology. General reflexology to support the system.
Some problems	A definition of the problem. Simple physiology of how the problem may have occurred. Suggested reflexology to include in a reflexology session.
Reflex zones	When part of the anatomy is named in the reflexology therapy tables please assume it is the foot reflex zone unless otherwise stated.

MAMMARY SYSTEM

Breasts	Breasts are always responsive to the effects of hormones. Throughout pregnancy mammary tissue was laid down and colostrum produced. Now the breasts prepare for breast-feeding.
Metaphysical aspects	The breasts are the organs of nurturing.
Reflexology	Encourage and maintain normal function. Acknowledge the nurturing and loving aspects.

LACTATION

During pregnancy some of the pregnancy hormones stimulate the breasts to produce colostrum. Colostrum is packed with nutrients and has little fluid volume - the baby is well hydrated in utero and therefore needs very little fluid during the first few days. The trigger for milk production is the lack of placental hormones; the mother's milk "comes in" on about the third day after birthing. Constant sucking by the baby encourages an earlier start to lactation. Pain, tension, stress, emotional upheaval, performance anxiety, maternal illness, traumatic labour, timed feedings and poor attachment to the breast can delay the lactation process and inhibit the let down reflex, making the milk less available.

Reflexology	
Endocrine system	Balance - to promote the natural energies of lactation.
Breasts	Massage - to encourage loving, nurturing emotions and pleasure.
Chest and lungs	Fish, dolphin - to maintain relaxation.

BREAST ENGORGEMENT

Immediately prior to the milk "coming in" the breasts have an increase in the blood supply - engorgement.

Reflexology	
Breasts, direct	Thumb walk - to relieve discomfort. Massage - to encourage suppleness.
Breasts, direct and indirect	Linking between both breast zones - to balance the energy.
Axillary lymphatics	Lymphatic technique - to assist removal of excess fluid.
"Solar plexus"	Bimanual hold - to ease anxiety.

LACTATION, UNDER SUPPLY, SLOW LET DOWN REFLEX AND FAILURE TO LACTATE

Reflexology	
Pituitary	Stimulate - to encourage milk production.
Nipple and pituitary	Link - to encourage milk flow.
Breasts	Stimulate - to increase milk production.
Chest / breast	Loosening relaxations: fish, dolphin, flip flops, metatarsal stretch, thumb slide, fist slide - to relax the area and reduce tension.
Shoulders and neck	Gentle flip flops, fish and dolphin - to relax the area.

Note

It has been observed that clients who have had an IVI sited in the back of the hand - the hand indirect breast reflex zone - may have delayed lactation.

LACTATION, OVER SUPPLY AND RAPID LET DOWN REFLEX

Reflexology	
Endocrine system	Endocrine balance - to balance.

What Elsa says

"Reassure the client that things will settle down after a few days."

SUPPRESSION OF LACTATION

Lactation works on a supply and demand basis. Stimulation of the breast by baby's sucking produces the hormones to supply the amount of milk required by the baby. The more the baby sucks, the more milk is made. If lactation is to be suppressed it is important to NOT STIMULATE the breasts. There are occasions when it is not possible to breast-feed the baby, for example, if the mother does not want to or is unable to. The reasons may be physical or emotional. The baby may not be able to feed due to immaturity, illness, death or adoption. Sometimes the baby will refuse to breast-feed.

Reflexology	
"Solar plexus"	Bimanual hold - to lessen anxiety.
Lymphatic system	Lymphatic technique - to help the body remove excess fluid.
Urinary system	Flush - to help the body excrete excess fluid.

Caution — **Do NOT stimulate the breast reflection zones**

What Elsa says

"Support the client's choice to suppress lactation and / or give TLC+++ if the choice was not made by her. Be empathic. Women who have wanted to breast-feed and are unable to, or who have enjoyed breast-feeding and now need to wean the baby will suffer some degree of loss and therefore grief when suppressing lactation."

MASTITIS

Mastitis is inflammation of part or the entire breast and is often caused by a blocked milk-duct.

Reflexology	
Breasts	Direct and indirect zones, gently massage the direction the milk ducts flow - to ease the pain and loosen lumps and blockages.
Axillary lymphatics	Lymphatic technique, with special attention to axillary lymphatics - to promote removal of cell debris and encourage cell health.
The centre of the mastitis	*If possible trigger point - to clear blockages and hasten healing.
Caution	***This will be painful**

NIPPLE TENDERNESS / TRAUMA

Nipple care routines change frequently, often causing confusion for the mother. Current trends recommend that hind milk is the only substance used for routine nipple care. Commercial products such as lotions and creams should be avoided as they dry the nipples and interfere with the mother's natural scent which is so important for bonding and baby learning tastes and smells. Some nipple tenderness is normal in the postnatal period, as nipples tend to be extra sensitive during pregnancy.

Reflexology	
Nipple	Sedate - to ease pain.
Breast	Sedate - to ease tension.
Breast / chest	Relaxations: fish, dolphin - to encourage the flow of energy.

What Elsa says *"Advise the client to seek sound lactation advice e.g. good attachment techniques."*

BREAST-FEEDING FOR THOSE MUMS ABOUT TO QUIT

Sometimes it is difficult to realise that breast-feeding is a natural activity. It can be frustrating, painful, exhausting and downright horrible! Mums get different advice from the professionals. Sometimes mum knows how to do it and sometimes the baby knows. One way and another it can be easy to quit. Someone has to believe that it is worthwhile in the end.

Reflexology	
Longitudinal zones	Brazilian Balance - to balance the entire being.
Diaphragm	Pivot across - to help to get through those really trying and emotional moments when it all seems too difficult to continue breast feeding.
"Solar plexus"	Bimanual hold - to give time to debrief and regain sense of self-worth.
Heart	Calming hold - to nurture.
Lungs	Metatarsal stretch and lung press - to help overcome feelings of sadness and grief.

What Elsa says *"Whatever mum decides is OK."*

MUSCULOSKELETAL SYSTEM

ACHING JOINTS AND MUSCLES

A strenuous active birthing can cause aches from the tip of the nose to the tip of the toes! The physiology is the same as taking any extreme physical exercise - the muscles get stiff. After giving birth and for the duration of breast-feeding low oestrogen levels cause menopausal-like symptoms such as aching joints. The pelvic joints and ligaments take about three months to return to being a solid structure.

Reflexology	
Entire body	Relaxation all - to relieve the aches.
Endocrine system	Balance - to help restore a non pregnant hormonal balance.

What Elsa says *"Reassure the client that this is a normal condition that will improve once her menstrual cycles return."*

DIASTASIS RECTI ABDOMINIS

The abdominal muscles usually regain their tone in a few months. Diastases recti abdominis is a condition where the long muscles of the abdomen separate at the mid-line. It is more likely to occur in women who have had several pregnancies or a multiple birth.

Reflexology	
Abdomen	Stimulate - to increase vitality to region.
Spine	Stimulate - to strengthen while abdomen is not aiding support to the back.
Note	This treatment is in addition to any physiotherapy exercises.

REPRODUCTIVE SYSTEM

INVOLUTION

Involution is the term given to the process of the reproductive system regaining its non-pregnant state and preparing for its non-pregnant function - menstrual cycles. It usually takes six to eight weeks.

Reflexology	
Entire body	Full reflexology sessions.

INVOLUTION OF THE UTERUS

Nature has designed the uterus to continue contracting after birth. This amazing organ, which during pregnancy increased 2,200% in size, now has ten days to regain its non-pregnant size, shape and position in the pelvis.

Reflexology	
Abdomen	Wind screen wipers and strong fist slide - to encourage abdominal activity.
Internal pelvis	Massage - to promote health.

AFTER-PAINS

After-pains are uterine contractions caused by the involution of the uterus. These can continue for up to seven days after delivery. Many first time mothers are oblivious to these contractions but mothers having their second and subsequent babies will experience painful contractions that are hugely aggravated by breast-feeding.

Reflexology	
Uterus	Healing hold - to acknowledge its pain.
"Solar plexus"	Bimanual hold - to restore calm.
Hips	Ankle boogie - to ease hip cramp.
Shoulder girdle	Relaxations: fish and dolphin - to relax the rest of the body.
Spine	Spinal twist - to loosen tension in the spine.

Caution

**The uterus reflex zones are meant to be well contracted.
Do NOT relax them.**

What Elsa says

"Explain to the client why these contractions are occurring. Knowing that they are normal and beneficial and of limited duration may help her tolerate the discomfort."

SUBINVOLUTION OF THE UTERUS

Within ten days after birthing the uterus should be entirely in the pelvis and by six weeks should have involuted to its non-pregnant size. Infection, retained fragments of placenta and membranes and an overstretched or exhausted uterus can all lead to poor contractility of the uterine muscle and hence poor involution of the uterus.

Reflexology	
Uterus	Firmly stimulate - to energise the area. Double thumb walk from abdomen to pelvis - to encourage uterine contraction.
Caution  	**Before commencement be sure to warn the client that this technique can be quite painful.**

LOCHIA

Lochia is the vaginal discharge that occurs after birthing. For the first few days it is red and copious, it then turns brown and slight, then pinkish and scant, then fades away.

Reflexology	
Abdomen & pelvis	Stimulate - to maintain the normal healthy process.

OFFENSIVE LOCHIA

Lochia has a distinctive smell, which is not unpleasant. The smell of lochia becomes offensive when there is a problem, which is often caused by infection or retained fragments of placenta and membranes.

Reflexology	
Uterus	Firmly stimulate - to encourage contraction and passing of clots and placental debris.
"Solar plexus"	Bimanual hold - to ease anxiety.
Thymus	Tap - to boost the immune system.
Lymphatic system	Lymphatic technique - to remove toxins.

Caution

This is an obstetric problem and needs professional care.

PERINEAL PAIN

The birthing process can be traumatic to the tissues of the vagina and perineum. During the second stage of labour contractions forced the baby onto the pelvic floor muscles causing a certain amount of bruising and swelling. The vaginal opening is stretched thin, sometimes tearing to allow more space for the emerging baby. An episiotomy may have been performed to aid the birth. Stitches to repair a tear or episiotomy increase the discomfort. Perineal pain / discomfort is likely to increase during the first three or four days after the birth gradually diminishing from then on. This area should be healed within about six weeks. After six weeks slight tenderness around the scarred area is quite normal with intimate physical contact. Vaginal dryness whilst breast-feeding and tension if fearing pain will accentuate the tenderness.

Reflexology

Perineum	Sedate - to ease the pain. Healing hold - to encourage tissue repair.
Pelvic lymphatics	Stimulate - to help remove damaged cells and promote cell regeneration.
Lymphatic system	Lymphatic technique - to promote removal of cell debris.
Urinary system	"Flush" - to help excrete fluid waste.

ALIMENTARY SYSTEM

While the body is birthing it does not do digesting! Throughout her labour the client would have eaten nothing or very little. Many women feel starving hungry after birthing. (The author wonders if this is a throwback to the times when all mammals including humans ate the placenta). Some women feel nauseated and vomit.

Reflexology

The whole system	The whole alimentary system - to regain its tone.

NORMAL BOWEL MOVEMENT

At birth the bowels are empty. It takes a few days for them to be fully functional again.

Reflexology

Abdomen	Wind screen wipers, strong fist slide - to encourage abdominal activity.
Large intestine	Thumb walk the direction of the flow - to promote vitality.
Rectum	Thumb walk and massage - to promote vitality.

CONSTIPATION

Immediately prior to birthing the woman will naturally empty her bowels, which may be diarrhoea-like. During birthing the contents of the rectum will be expelled. After delivery several days may pass without the woman having her bowels open. If there has been perineal trauma there will be a great reluctance to defecate and constipation will develop.

Reflexology	
Large intestine	Stimulate - to increase energy to the area. Massage using the direction of the flow - to reinstate the energy direction.
Anus	Sedate - to ease pain and fear.
Spine	Spinal twist and spine stretches - to relax the whole area especially the lower back.
Hips	Ankle boogie and ankle rotations - to ease the tension.

What Elsa says

"It may take time to retrain the bowels after childbirth. Advise the client to only push gently when having her bowels open. Use aperients with caution as they may affect the breast fed baby."

HAEMORRHOIDS

Haemorrhoids are varicosed veins of the rectum and anus.

Straining to push during the second stage of labour, a long second stage of labour, large baby and instrumental deliveries are probable causes.

If the problem is not resolved in the early days after birthing it may persist for several months and even become chronic.

Reflexology	
Anus	Sedate - to ease pain and fear. If possible trigger point release - to remove the blocked energy.
Spine	Spinal twist and spine stretches - to relax the whole area especially the lower back.
Hips	Ankle boogie and ankle rotations - to ease the tension.
Pelvic lymphatics	Stimulate - to promote removal of cell debris.

URINARY SYSTEM

MICTURITION (passing urine)

Within an hour of giving birth the kidneys re-set the fluid balance and most women void a huge quantity of urine (diuresis).

Reflexology

Urinary system	"Flush" - to encourage normal action.

DYSURIA, DIFFICULTY WITH MICTURITION AND FAILURE TO MICTURATE

Dysuria is painful micturition.

Reflexology First Aid

Internal pelvis	Sedate and healing hold - to ease the tension.
Urinary system	"Flush" - to restore the integrity of the urinary system.
Bladder	Stimulate - to regain the energy to function well and restore the tone.
Urethra	Sedate - to ease the pain.
Internal pelvis	Sedate - to ease the tension.
Pelvic nerves	Normalise - to help restore good function.
Hips	Gentle ankle boogie and ankle rotations - to relax the area.

Note

It is very important that after any of the above the bladder needs to regain its tone. If the bladder tone is poor the client may suffer stress incontinence, which may last for many years.

STRESS INCONTINENCE

Stress incontinence is the involuntary passing of small amounts of urine. It is caused from trauma during birthing. It may be temporary or continue for many years. This problem shows up when coughing and sneezing.

Reflexology

Bladder	Strongly stimulate - to help regain tone.

Note

Teach the client how to stimulate bladder reflex zones.
To know if the bladder tone is good the "edge " of the bladder reflex zone feels more defined.

CARDIOVASCULAR SYSTEM

Blood volume	The hypervolaemia that was experienced during pregnancy will naturally resolve with the blood loss during birthing and the lochia.
Blood clotting	The blood no longer needs its extra clotting ability and returns to normal.
Blood pressure	The blood pressure returns to its non-pregnant levels.

Reflexology	
Entire body	Full reflexology session.

RECOVERY FROM POST PARTUM HAEMORRHAGE (PPH)

A post partum haemorrhage will make the client feel tired and lethargic. PPH is an obstetric emergency and the client will have experienced great anxiety.

Reflexology	
Uterus	Firmly stimulate - to provide energy to contract.
Spleen	Gently stimulate - to encourage blood health and assist the immune system.
Liver	Gently stimulate - to encourage blood health.
Heart	Moderately stimulate - to promote joy.
"Solar plexus"	Bimanual hold - to reduce anxiety and distress and reinstate the life-force.
Spleen	Stimulate - to promote spleen vitality.

Caution

This is NOT instead of obstetric emergency procedures for PPH. This reflexology treatment is for the recovery phase.

DEEP VEIN THROMBOSIS (DVT)

DVT is a major medical problem. The client will be under medical supervision for a long time.

Contraindication

REFLEXOLOGY CONTRAINDICATED

STOP

Note

Once the medical problem is resolved, reflexology therapy may be resumed.

VARICOSE VEINS OF THE LEGS

Varicose veins of the legs are surface veins with weakened walls, which allow a ballooning effect of the blood vessel. They may be asymptomatic but are likely to ache, be painful, look unsightly and may even hinder daily activities. Pregnancy tends to worsen existing varicosities and increase the risk of developing new ones. Most pregnancy-induced varicosities improve during the postnatal period but are unlikely to return to normal and continue to be problematic.

Reflexology

Varicose vein	Referral areas thumb walk - to encourage healing.
Internal pelvis	*Trigger Point Release - to clear blocked energy.
Pelvic lymphatics	Stimulate - to encourage vitality.

*To locate the exact zone gently palpate the internal pelvic reflex zones. The area, which is exquisitely tender, is very probably the reflex of where the original energy blockage occurred.

LYMPHATIC SYSTEM

After birthing the lymphatic system removes waste products left over from the pregnancy and any damaged cells caused by the birthing.

Reflexology

The entire system	Reflexology lymphatic technique - to support the natural process.

OEDEMA

Oedema is excess interstitial fluid. It is more commonly a pregnancy condition though some women who do not have it during pregnancy then develop it after birthing.

Reflexology

Lymphatic system	Lymphatic technique - to assist removal of excess fluid.
Urinary system	"Flush" - to support the lymphatic technique.

RESPIRATORY SYSTEM

The lungs are no longer squashed and the client can breathe freely again!

Reflexology	
Chest and lungs	Full chest routine.

AFTER GENERAL ANAESTHETIC

Reflexology	
Lymphatic system	Lymphatic technique - to assist the removal of toxins.
Liver	Stimulate - to assist the removal of toxins.
Thymus	Tap - to boost the immune system.
"Solar plexus"	Bimanual hold - to reduce anxiety and fear.
Lungs	Lung press - to encourage removal of poisonous gasses.

NERVOUS SYSTEM

Pelvic nerves — The pelvic nerves - bowel and bladder nerves - may take several months after birthing to send unscrambled information to the brain.

Sexual nerves — The nerves that pick up sexual pleasure may take anything from six weeks to several years to regain normality.

Reflexology	
Entire body	Relaxation techniques - to promote healing.

AFTER EPIDURAL ANAESTHESIA

Epidural anaesthesia can provide total pain control from the site of the epidural to the feet. Many women choose to use this anaesthetic during labour and for Caesarean Section. After the birth the anaesthetic takes two to three hours to wear off. Women may experience tingling in their legs, headaches and backaches, which may last for a long time.

Reflexology	
Site of epidural (lumbar vertebrae)	*Trigger Point Release (see page 159) - to clear the blocked energies created by the epidural.
Spine	Gentle spinal twists - to relax the spine and promote re-establishment of energy flow.
Pelvis	Gentle ankle boogie - to restore energy to the pelvis and hips.
Coccyx and head	Linking - to rebalance the spine.

SCIATIC PAIN

Sciatic pain may be caused by the involution of the ligaments of the pelvis. It is more common in women who have had C/S.

Reflexology	
Hips and pelvis	Relaxation - to ease the tension.
Greater sciatic notch	Trigger point release - to clear blocked energies.

TENSION HEADACHES

Tension headaches are frequently caused by the responsibility of being a new mother and not yet knowing how to understand a newborn baby.

Reflexology	
Entire body	All relaxation techniques - to reduce the tension.
Head and neck	Toe stretches and rotations - to relieve the tension.
Spine	Spinal twist and very gentle spine runs - to release back tension.
Diaphragm	Pivot across - to release emotional energies.

EXHAUSTION, FATIGUE

The weeks and months following birthing can be exhausting - a confusion of emotions both welcome and unwelcome and the physical strain a new baby inflicts on all the family. Recuperation from the birth is hindered by broken night-time sleep patterns and the household running of washing, feeding the family, receiving visitors and minimising sibling rivalry.

Reflexology	
Entire body	Relaxation - all very slowly and gently - to encourage rest, relaxation and recuperation.
Longitudinal zones	"Brazilian Balance" - to realign the body's energies.
"Solar plexus"	Hold - to calm and settle.

Note Exhaustion and fatigue may last for years and undermine the woman's health, wellbeing, her ability to cope and so on.

INTEGUMENTARY SYSTEM

The skin

The abdominal skin that has been so stretched takes about three months to regain its tone.

STRETCH MARKS

Stretch marks may develop during pregnancy. They can be slight and pink or even extensive and purple.

Reflexology

Abdomen, breasts, hips and thighs	Massage - to nurture.
Entire body	All relaxation techniques - to help her accept the status quo.

What Elsa says

"It is a great sadness to many women that stretch marks will never disappear. They will fade but never go. There are no ways to remove stretch marks; help the client come to terms with them."

ENDOCRINE SYSTEM

No placenta

After the delivery of the placenta there are no placental hormones. The levels of the hormones of pregnancy decline and are not replaced. The client feels withdrawal symptoms, also known as the "third day blues".

Lactation hormones

The hormones of lactation come into effect immediately after birthing.

Fertility hormones

The hormones of fertility kick-in at about six weeks after birthing.

Ovaries

Without the effects of the hormones of pregnancy the ovaries are stimulated to produce oestrogen and progesterone and recommence the menstrual cycles.

Remember: ovulation occurs before menstruation. Which means that the woman may conceive without first having a menstrual period.

Reflexology

Endocrine system	Endocrine balance - to support the natural process.

DIABETES AND GESTATIONAL DIABETES

Caution

Diabetic women return to their non-pregnant diabetic management immediately after birthing. At this time diabetic clients are especially unstable and must have medical supervision. Gestational diabetes will no longer exist after birthing.

Reflexology

Endocrine system	Endocrine balance several times - to help the body adjust to different hormone requirements.
Pancreas	Gently stimulate - to support the different insulin requirement.
Liver	Stimulate - to support its heavy work load.

PSYCHOLOGICAL ASPECTS

Emotions	Major emotional changes happen to women after birthing. It takes about three months for many women to feel "normal" again.
Emotional lability	During the early postnatal days emotional lability is very common.

THIRD DAY BLUES

On about day three after birthing the mother will probably become weepy. Often there is no obvious reason for the tears, although sore nipples, sleeplessness and the responsibility of motherhood may contribute to the emotional seesaw.

The third day blues are due to hormonal changes after the birth and usually subside over 24 to 48 hours.

The third day blues are a natural reaction and occur after about 80% of births.

Reflexology

Entire body	Relaxations all - to help experience the experience of early motherhood.
Endocrine system	Balance - to help the client's body accept the absence of placental hormones.
"Solar plexus"	Bimanual hold - to settle emotions.
Balance organ and "Sense of Self"	Link - to help establish the new self.

POSTNATAL DEPRESSION

Postnatal depression (PND) should not be confused with the "blues" or puerperal psychosis, both of which occur very soon after birthing. PND is not usually diagnosed until the baby is over six weeks old. Prior to this, depression is usually related to sleep deprivation. The cause of PND was thought to be from hormonal changes after birthing; this belief is now being questioned as both men and women suffer from PND. Some experts suggest that PND should be thought of as post traumatic stress in that the total change in lifestyle and the burden of parenthood is traumatic and this trauma leads to depression. Whatever the cause, being depressed is a very real situation; sufferers cannot "just snap out of it". PND is not "just put on" for attention. Men and women with PND should seek professional help rather than trying to put on a brave face or struggle on unsupported.

Reflexology

Entire body	Relaxations all - to help to "go with the flow" and get a good nights sleep.
"Solar plexus"	Bimanual hold - to calm and settle.
Balance organ and "Sense of Self"	Link - to help find the self.
Spine	Spinal twist, rubs and runs - to promote energy flow.
Uterus, indirect ovary, "solar plexus" and hypothalamus	Link - to balance bottom, middle and top.
Longitudinal zones	"Brazilian Balance" - to straighten out the kinks in the longitudinal energy.

What Elsa says	*"Help the parents to differentiate between sleep deprivation and PND. Encourage them to seek help."*

POST TRAUMATIC STRESS, DIFFICULT OR TRAUMATIC DELIVERY, UNEXPECTED OUTCOME OR EMOTIONALLLY TRAUMATIC DELIVERY

Until it is over no one knows how birthing will affect the mother. Birthing is an enormous experience and different personalities will perceive it differently. Some mothers are very traumatised by the whole experience.

Reflexology	
Entire body	Relaxations all - to nurture and show empathy and give time to debrief.
"Solar plexus"	Bimanual hold - to ease distress.
Chest	Lung press, metatarsal stretch, fish, dolphin - to calm and settle and help overcome feelings of loss and grief.
Diaphragm	Pivot across - to release agitation and emotions.
Longitudinal zones	Brazilian Balance - to balance the entire being.

RESTRICTED CONTACT WITH BABY

There may be times when mother and baby are parted. This runs against the mother's instincts to be with her baby and may have long term affect on their relationship. If there is restricted contact with the baby it is probably due to some problem, such as mother or baby are unwell.

Reflexology	
Entire body	General loving touch - to nurture and to boost when feeling depressed.
Lungs	Metatarsal stretch and lung press - to acknowledge feelings of sadness and loss.
Diaphragm	Pivot along - to release tension and emotions.
"Solar plexus"	Bimanual hold - to calm and settle.

MOTHER AND BABY SEPERATED: ILL BABY, DECEASED BABY, BABY FOR ADOPTION

These are dreadful times for the mother and cause much soul searching and grief.

Reflexology	
Entire body	General loving touch - to nurture and to boost when feeling distressed and depressed.

Note

Use your most exquisite listening skills and your heart-felt attitude of relatedness, connectedness and beingness.

Be sure to take care of yourself.

Reflexology Techniques

TRIGGER POINT RELEASE

The reflexology Trigger Point Release is one of reflexology techniques used to move blockages. This technique is excellent for clearing localised blockage of energy.

GENERAL INFORMATION

The Trigger Point Release	The Trigger Point Release is a very powerful technique that moves blocked energies with force.
Use with care	It needs to be used with great care and only when absolutely necessary, for example, after an epidural or when the blocked energy will not move using other techniques.
Client consent	This technique is very effective but is extremely unpleasant for the client. It is necessary to have full informed consent.
Note	When the client displays pain or great discomfort, reassure her that it is expected.
Important	Once this technique is started it is important to continue till the end. DO NOT release the grip, or pain will have been inflicted on the client without the therapeutic benefit.
Once only	If there is a strong reaction to the trigger point release use it once only during a reflexology session.
Practical reminder	To do this technique the reflexologists must have very short thumbnails.

Method

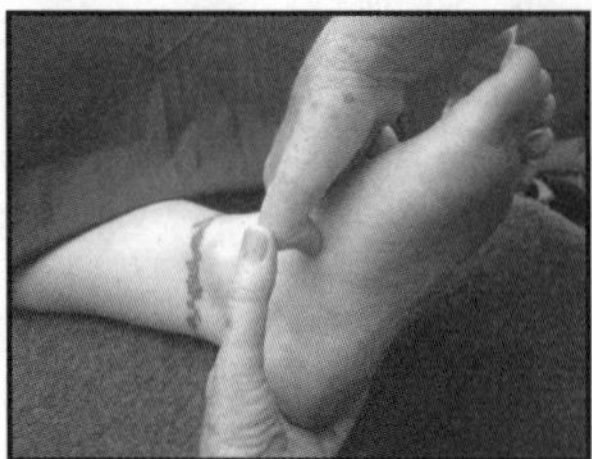

Thumb or finger walk to locate the epicentre of the disordered zone. Ask the client to confirm the exact area.

Using the thumb at a right angle (90°) press deeply into the zone.

Maintain the pressure for up to two minutes.

If necessary support the working thumb with the thumb of the other hand.

To release the hold take the pressure off slowly.

How to know when to release

After the great rush of energy to the reflex zone, the hurting sensation eases for the client.
As the reflex zone regains its vitality the reflexologist can feel wriggling type sensation under his/her thumb.
The wriggling then becomes a pulsing - a therapeutic pulse - not a heartbeat pulse.

CLIENT RESPONSE

Client response

When the trigger point is first applied the client often feels a rush of energy (pain) to the area, then a surge of energy up her body.

Precaution
The "Oh Shit" reaction

The client response is usually vocal and can surprise the client and the practitioner.

Stoic

Some clients are stoic and suppress a noisy reaction.

Flash back

Sometimes clients experience a flash back to when the disorder first happened. This can cause a cathartic reaction.

REFLEXOLOGIST RESPONSE

Cathartic reaction

If there is a cathartic reaction it can be frightening for both client and practitioner.

Empathic response

An empathic response, such as listening to the client in a non-prejudicial and non-judgemental way. It may have been many years the hurt has been buried.

EXPECTED OUTCOME

On many occasions after a trigger point release the disorder does not recur.

Postnatal Care for the Baby

It is noticeable that one of the first things that a mother does after her baby is born is to check his/her toes. Could it be some instinctual knowing about the significance of toes?

It is always delicious to kiss a newborn baby's toes. Encourage the mother to do so - it will send such good messages to the baby. Show the mother "hullo feet", loving and playful movements and special times between mother and baby. These are wonderful beginnings to a life with reflexology!

Blood tests

Between six and fourteen days after birth babies are screened for several medical problems.
Blood is taken from the baby by a heel prick.

Reflexology significance

This is usually an unpleasant experience for the baby who may become wary of having his/her feet touched again.

SIMPLE REFLEXOLOGY FOR THE PARENTS

GENERAL INFORMATION

Reflexology

Reflexology is such an uncomplicated modality. It is easy to understand, easy to do and effective.

A blessing

It is such a blessing for new parents to have something at their fingertips that is both pleasurable for the baby and can help minor problems of infancy.

The following information is to give the reflexologist some ideas of how to share their skills with the parents.

What is reflexology?

Give a simple definition of reflexology, which is easily understandable.

When to "do" reflexology

Whenever it takes the mum's or dad's fancy is a good time to "do" reflexology.

Some good times are:

- Before bed-time.
- "Hello its nice to see you again" after rest time.
- Play time - "This little piggie went to market" is a fun game.
- Bath time.
- When "scary things happen" time.
- Minor problems time.

How long to "do" reflexology

"Read" the signals given by the baby to know how long to "do" reflexology. Some times half a minute is long enough and sometimes ten minutes is not long enough.

How to position a baby

There are many ways to position a baby for reflexology:

- When breast feeding.
- Lying on the lap with feet towards mum / dad.
- On the changing table, pram, high chair or similar.

Bigger babies can be carried on the hip - do one foot, change to the other hip and do the other foot.

Even bigger babies - try sitting on dad's shoulders.

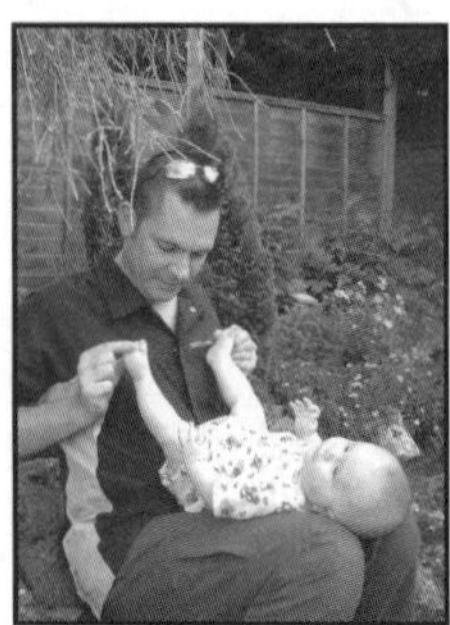

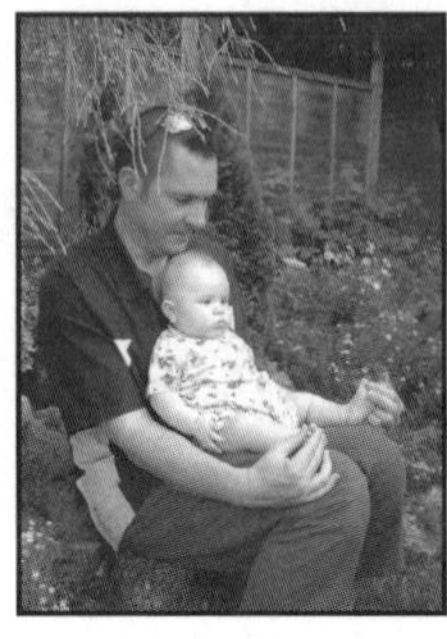

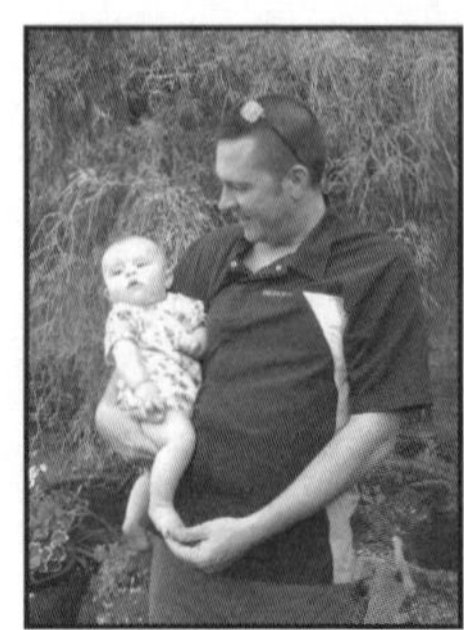

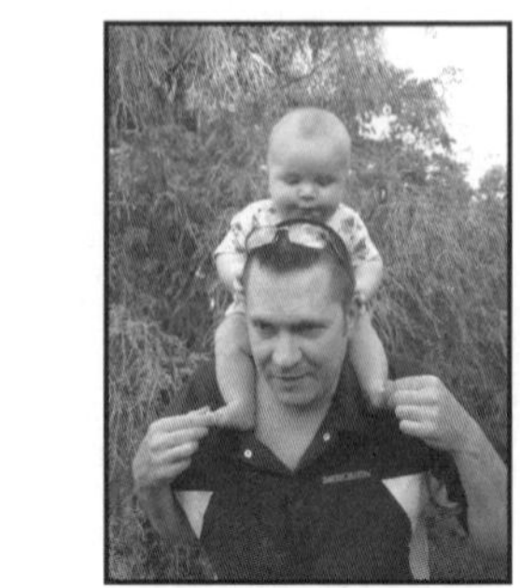

What pressure to use

Usually use a fairly light pressure. Judge by whether it tickles or not. (Tickling for a baby can be a form of pain and his squealing may not be delight but dread).

HAPPY CONTENTED BABIES

Reflexology

Entire body	General loving technique, kiss toes and feet, "hullo feet" - to welcome baby to this world and his family.
Shoulder girdle	Flip-flops - to enjoy mum's company and have fun.

BABIES WITH "TUMMY" ACHES

COLIC

Colic is an abdominal pain, which may be caused by indigestion or "wind".

Reflexology

Abdomen	Bimanual "solar plexus" hold - to calm. Wind screen wipers - to move the discomfort. Wind up and wind down - to balance normal digestive function.
Coping point	Hold - to help settle.
"Solar plexus"	Hold - to calm.

POSITING

Positing is when babies vomit small quantities frequently with no apparent reason.

Reflexology

Digestive tract	Massage along the direction of the "flow" - to encourage peristalsis.

GASTRO-OESOPHAGEAL REFLUX

Gastro-oesophageal reflux is a condition where the acid stomach contents enter the oesophagus - it is very painful.

Reflexology

Stomach	Sedate - to help prevent over-activity.
"Solar plexus"	Bimanual thumb hold - to calm and relieve tension / fear.
Oesophagus	Sedate - to relieve pain.

VOMITING

Occasional vomiting for a baby is a normal occurrence; however if the vomiting is copious, projectile and frequent the parents must seek medical attention.

Reflexology	
Stomach	Sedate - to settle the stomach.
"Solar plexus"	Bimanual hold - to allay anxiety and fear.

CONSTIPATION

Constipation is the passing of infrequent, hard stools. Breast fed babies are rarely constipated. If the problem persists advise the parents to seek baby care advice on feeding.

Reflexology	
Abdomen	Tiny fist slide - to encourage peristalsis.
Large intestine	Stimulate - to energise the bowel. Massage the direction of flow - to encourage peristalsis.
Hips	Ankle boogie and ankle rotations - to loosen up and take the tension from the hips.
Spine	Gentle spinal twist - to release tension.

What Elsa says

"This treatment is much more gentle than laxatives and more effective than changing from one brand of formula to another and back again."

BABIES WITH HEADACHES

UNSETTLED BABIES, CRYING AND WITH PAIN CAUSING HEADACHES

Reflexology	
Heart	Calming hold - to calm and settle the spirit.
"Solar plexus"	Bimanual (or one at a time) hold - to counteract fear and shock.
Head	Very gentle toe stretches and rotations - to ease tension.
Diaphragm	Pivot across diaphragm - to release emotional energies.
Big toe	Hold - to encourage endorphin release.
Spine	Spinal twist and stretch - to ease back tension Feather light spine runs - to clear energy flow.

Note

Headaches are included as any baby crying for extended periods is bound to end up with a tension headache!

OVERACTIVE BABIES

CRYING, EMOTIONAL DISTRESS, ANGRY BABIES

Reflexology	
"Solar plexus"	Bimanual hold - to calm and settle anxiety.
Entire body	General loving - to nurture and share the experience. Relaxations yin/yang and dolphin - to gentle the distress.
Longitudinal zones	Brazilian Balance (a form of "this little piggie) to move blockages from the energy channels congested by crying.
Heart	Calming hold - to settle the spirit.
Lungs	Lung press - to calm respirations.
Head	Sedate - to encourage endorphin release.

IRRITABLE & HIGHLY STRUNG BABIES

Reflexology	
Entire body	Calming hold - to reduce stress and tension.
Muscles	Relaxation: dolphin - to reduce muscle tension and resultant fatigue.
"Solar plexus"	Bimanual hold - to calm and settle anxiety.

What Elsa says

"For those times when all the physical needs are met and baby is still asking for help. The above techniques will lower the frustration and hopelessness experienced at times by the mum."

UNDERACTIVE BABIES

POOR FEEDER, SLEEPY BABY

Reflexology	
Spine	Spine runs (up) - to stimulate.

SPECIAL CARE BABIES

Some babies begin their life needing special care in hospital. Babies born pre-term or babies who are unwell fall into this category. A form of reflexology that is extremely light may be used. It is known to be of help to both the baby and his/her parents. This form of reflexology is too specialised to be included in this text. However several reflexologists and special care midwives / nurses are developing this form of care.

Recommended reading for parents who have a baby in the special care nursery *Reflexology a Tool for Midwives,* chapter 7 *"Reflexology and Premature Babies"* contributed by Helen Croser.

Appendices

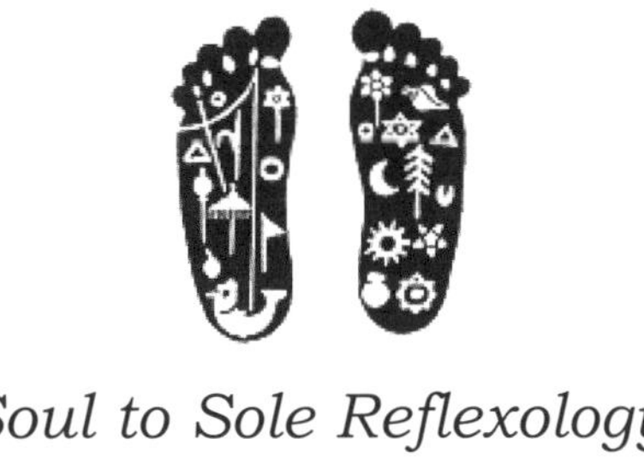

Soul to Sole Reflexology

APPENDIX 1

CHINESE FOOT BINDING

Chinese foot-binding
Some comments

For the author the fascination of this custom is how did foot binding affect the women from the obstetric point of view? Obviously the next generation was conceived, carried throughout pregnancy and birthed - but knowing the effects of foot biomechanics on fertility and that everything in the feet is relayed to the being - how did it affect the women?

"Although the bound foot was described as aesthetically pleasing compared with the natural alternative, complications such as ulceration, paralysis and gangrene were not uncommon, and it has been estimated that as many as ten per cent of the girls did not survive the "treatment"." (Mackie G)

"Mothers impressed upon their daughters that the mark of a woman's attraction resided more in her character as revealed in the bind of her feet than in the face or body which nature had given her." (Blake C. F.)

"Women bound their feet to signify their claim on the dignity accorded those who embodied refinement and a "sense of class"." (Goody J)

"In a society with a cult of female chastity, one primary purpose of foot binding was to limit mobility, radically modifying the means by which females were permitted to become a part of the world at large." (Blake C. F.)

"Bound feet became a sexual fetish and were said to be conductive to better sexual intercourse." (Mackie G)

"A widespread male fantasy claimed that foot binding produced the development of a highly-muscled vagina full of wondrous folds." (Levy H. S)

APPENDIX 2

FROM INDIA

Contributed by Farida Irani
B.Com., D. Arom., DRT, DRM, D. Ref., D. Bow.

Feet of the Divine Mother

The feet of the Divine Mother and Father and the Gurus and Masters have been held in high reverence and touching the feet of the Divine Avatars and Gurus energises the devotee as the vibration received is of the highest form like a bolt of lightening.
When the devotee places her head at the feet of the master or mother the energy through the feet goes through the crown chakra into her entire being. It makes the devotee realise the magnanimity of the Cosmic Mother and the Masters thereby teaches her a lesson in humility as the Guru in turn blesses her by touching her head and balancing her chakras.

The Divine Mother

The different forms of the Divine Mother are all portrayed standing or sitting on a lotus, the Lotus symbolises purity and the chakras and therefore the feet of the Devine Mother and the Masters are always addressed as "lotus feet".
Devine Mother as Laxmi Goddess of prosperity and abundance is always in red and gold with gold coins pouring out of her hands and a beautiful lotus under her feet. As Saraswatti the divine aspect of wisdom and music she is holding a sitar in her hands. To think of the Divine Mother gives one a sense of being nurtured and loved.

The feet of a beech birth

A custom in India is that the feet of someone born in the breech position are considered to have healing properties and a kick from them will heal the receiver of the kick.

Ayurvedic foot massage
Padabhyanga

To keep a woman in a sweet disposition and to keep her dark moon times healthy, it is necessary daily to massage her feet with oil.
A daily foot massage, padabhyanga, is a simple and most revitalising sadhana for maintaining good health.
Padabhyanga has been practiced for millennia as a requisite to sound sleep, to infuse the day's activity with equanimity.
As a more exotic activity, in the royal courts of India and China padabhyanga has been used as a prelude to sexual activities.
According to Ayurveda, many marma points for the body's vital organs and sense organs are located in the soles of the feet.
Padabhyanga not only invigorates and renews the entire body but also encourages its natural "valium" to flow.
A peaceful night's rest or a calm day's activity is assured after the feet are thoroughly massaged."

Marma points of the foot

Kshipra Between the first and second toes.

Talhridaya Centre of the sole of the foot.

Kuruchcha Ball of the foot.

Kurchshira Heel and outer margin of the foot.

Gulpha Behind both sides of the ankle joint.

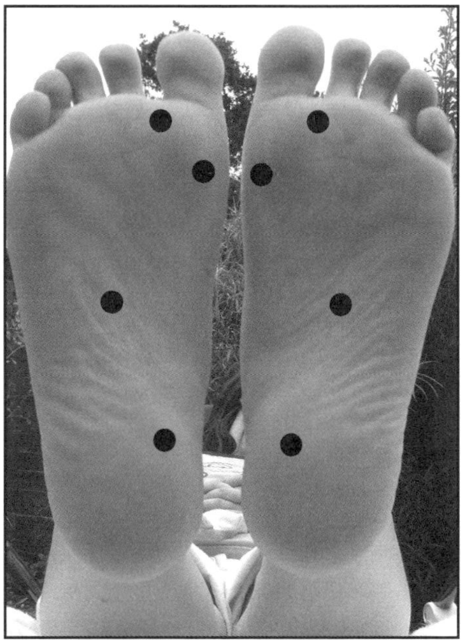

"Marma points are pressure points in the Ayurvedic system of massage occurring at the firm junctures of the five organic principles: sira (vessels), mansa (muscles), snayu (ligaments), asthi (bones) and sandhi (joints). These junctures form the seats of the vital life force or prana. At these junctures, the four classes of sira (vessels) - nerves, lymph, arteries and veins - enter the organism to carry nutrients and moisture to the muscles, ligaments, bones and joints." (Harishi Johari)

"By making a gentle circular movement with either the forefinger or middle finger on a marma, toxins can be released and eliminated by the body." (Sushruta Samhita)

"In Ayurvedic massage foot massage is included with the practices of massage, yoga asanas, pranayama and meditation, which affect the entire organism and promote optimum health of both body and mind. They unify the physical, emotional and spiritual sides of a pregnant woman, thus providing a better chemical environment for the growth of the child inside. These practices also enhance the likelihood of a quick recovery after childbirth." (Harishi Johari)

APPENDIX 3

BIOMECHANICS OF THE FEET AND PREGNANCY

Contributed by Jenny Devine M.A. Pod. A

Pregnancy creates significant alterations to posture and hence function of the feet. With a basic knowledge of biomechanics it is possible to assess the gait and gain insight into the health and well being of the client. Early recognition and interception of possible complications may assist in creating a comfortable pregnancy and an effective condition for a positive birth experience.

The modifications that occur in a woman's body during pregnancy are all part of the amazing process of birth. Apart from the obvious weight gain as the foetus develops, there are alterations in spinal alignment and increase in ligamentous laxity. All of these factors contribute to the typical stance and gait of a pregnant woman.

The gait

According to reflexology the five longitudinal zones should be stimulated via pressure during gait. The ideal gait consists of a heel strike on the lateral border (longitudinal zones 4-5); this is identified by the foot in a supinated position and with the ankle slightly dorsiflexed. As the ground contact continues, the foot moves rapidly into pronation with the lateral side of the forefoot making ground contact, and then the medial side of the forefoot is stimulated, with eventual "toe off". This propulsive action of walking has covered all five longitudinal zones.

During stance, a well-balanced foot should take pressure on all five longitudinal zones simultaneously. This will be reflected throughout the entire posture of the individual. An unsteady gait will create an unsteady structure. A pregnant woman with excessive subtalar joint pronation, genu valgum (knock knees), increased lumbar lordosis and flattening of the thoracic curve represents an unsteady structure.

In the client unsteady structure would result in her having painful feet, backache, she would tire easily and feel generally "off" balance.

The base of the gait

The base of the gait is the width between the medial maleoli during stance. Widening of the base has effects on gait stability and contributes to the typical "waddling" gait often observed in pregnant women. As the load increases, so does the need for stability.

"Widening the base of gait will increase the functional base of support during walking, producing a larger area in which the centre of mass can deviate from step to step". (Adam Bird).

An increased base of gait has *"the combined effect of directing body weight medial to the talus, producing excessive foot pronation and subsequent pathology"*. (William Root). This excessive pronation occurs at the talocalcaneal (subtalar joint) joint, which with **reference to reflexology** is the reflection for the sacro-iliac joint.

In the client this could result in her having lower back pain and aching hips. She may have feelings of instability and say, "I feel all at sea" and ungainliness and say "I feel like a beached whale".

Pronation

Pronation is a triplane action of the foot during motion. Pronation allows for the foot to become a loose structure when in contact with the ground, hence allowing for adaptation to various terrains and most importantly, shock absorption. This shock absorption mechanism is then relayed up to the knees, hips, pelvis and spine.
Excessive pronation is observed by a complete flattening of the medial arch during stance and not followed by any re-supination of the foot during motion. It indicates excessive strain on the sacro-iliac joint. This type of foot is likely to indicate a pelvis under stress.
With reference to reflexology this type of foot is likely to indicate a pelvis stressed by too much pressure. The structures and organs that lie in longitudinal zone 1 are stressed. This includes the spinal column, uterus, rectum and bladder.
The client with excessive pronation may have problems with constipation, menstrual cycles (dysmenorrhoea), dysuria, conceiving and birthing her baby. She may have feelings of keeping everything to herself and experience extreme privacy of her genital area. She may feel "flat" and unsupported.

Supination

Supination is a triplane action of the foot during motion. Supination makes the foot a rigid lever in preparation for toe off.
In excessive supination the rear foot may be observed from a posterior view and the calcaneus will be inverted, as indicated by the position of the Achillies tendon. A high arch, otherwise known as "pes cavus", indicates a foot like this.
With reference to reflexology this type of foot is likely to indicate a pelvis stressed by insufficient pressure.
If the foot were to be excessively supinated then the fifth longitudinal zone would be under stress.
The structures and organs in this zone that may be under stress are the shoulders, ascending and descending colons and perhaps the ovaries.
Clients with excessive supination may have problems with irregular menstrual cycles, retaining a conception, pre-term labour and precipitate deliveries.

Foot size

Another factor to take into consideration is the alteration in size of the feet during pregnancy. Usually the result of carrying an increased load combined with ligamentous laxity causes the feet to increase in length and width. This size alteration also remains during lactation.
Pregnant women need to be aware of this so that they do not squeeze their feet into their pre-pregnancy shoes and compromise blood supply to the feet.
In reference to reflexology; the feet reflect the alteration of the body structure of pregnancy and the increased breast size during lactation.
For the client, she would be well advised to not buy new shoes during pregnancy! During pregnancy most women are aware of the relief they obtain from comfortable footwear.

This brief piece will enhance awareness of the intricacy between foot function and its relationship with the rest of the body. A thorough observation of foot posture and gait will provide insights to assist the well being of the client.

Research

A Prospective Investigation of the Effects of Pregnancy on Footprint Parameters, Adam Bird et al, 1997

APPENDIX 4

REFLEXOLOGY ESTIMATION OF THE BONY PELVIS

This piece is taken from *Reflexology a Tool for Midwives,* 2002 by Susanne Enzer.

For interest

Although this technique is not necessary for reflexologists to know, it is included for interest.

Good question

Why do some midwives ask the shoe size of their pregnant clients?

Empiric knowledge

It is empiric knowledge that there is some correlation between the size of the feet and the pelvis - small feet small pelvis!
This is correct and reflexology can offer a precise way to assess the size and shape of the pelvis.

Adequate pelvis

Midwives need to have information about the shape, capacity and diameters of their client's pelvis to be sure that there will be no problem in the passageway for the birthing baby.

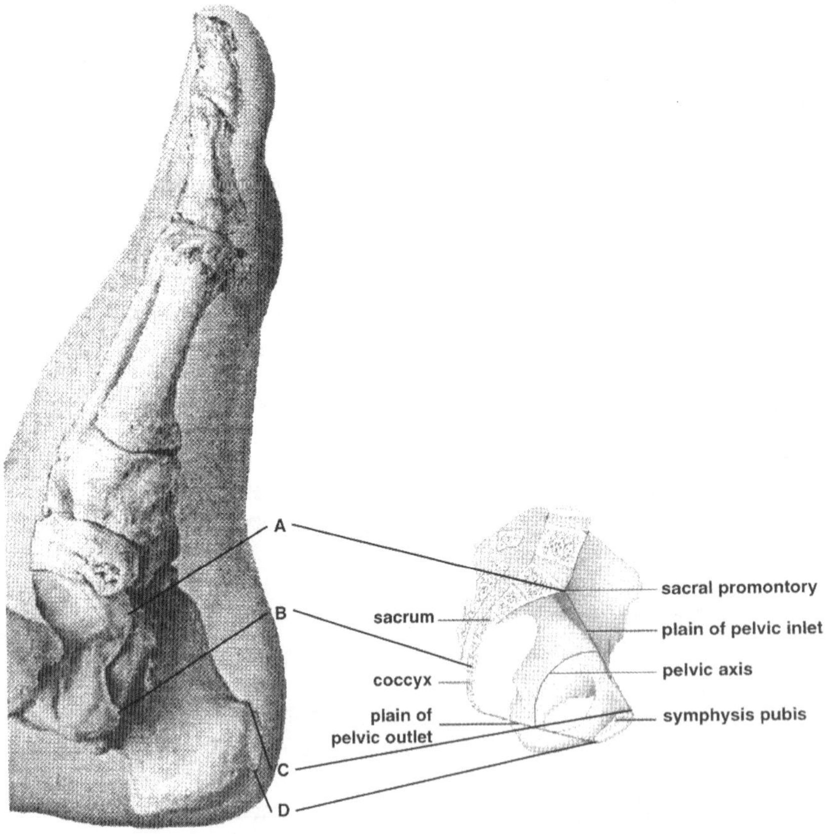

DIRECT SOMATIC REPLICATION (DSR)

Point A	DSR of the sacral promontory
Point B	DSR of the lower sacrum
Point C	DSR of the upper border of symphysis pubis
Point D	DSR of the lower inner border of symphysis pubis

Points A to B	DSR of the sacral curve
Points C to D	DSR of symphysis pubis
Points A to C	DSR of the pelvic inlet
Points B to D	DSR of the pelvic outlet

thod

Midwives need to know if the baby's head can get into the pelvis - the pelvic inlet. To turn around the baby needs a sacral curve that is neither too acute nor too flat. To get out the baby needs a good pelvic outlet and a sub-pubic arch of 90°.
Tell your fingers to feel bone not soft tissue.

cral curve

Using four fingers of one hand palpate the sub-talar joint. Points "A" to "B" on the diagram. Leave the fingers in position.
To assess the sacral curve observe the shape made by the fingers on the sub-talar joint. Whether it is well-defined or flat, long or short.

mphysis pubis

With the fingers of the other hand palpate the medial process of calcaneus. Points "C" to "D" on the diagram.

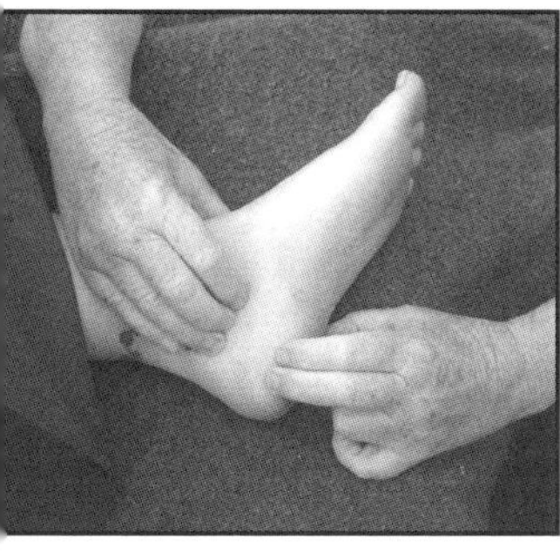

Keeping all fingers in place observe the relationship of the direct somatic replication of the sacral curve and symphysis pubis.

vic inlet

To assess the pelvic inlet estimate the distance between the fingers on points "A" and "C".

vic outlet

To assess the pelvic outlet estimate the distance between the fingers on points "B" and "D"

-pubic arch

To assess the sub-pubic arch hold the client's feet together under the ankles with one hand, raise the legs a little - sufficient to see the plantar aspect of the heels side by side. This is the direct somatic replication of the sub-pubic arch.

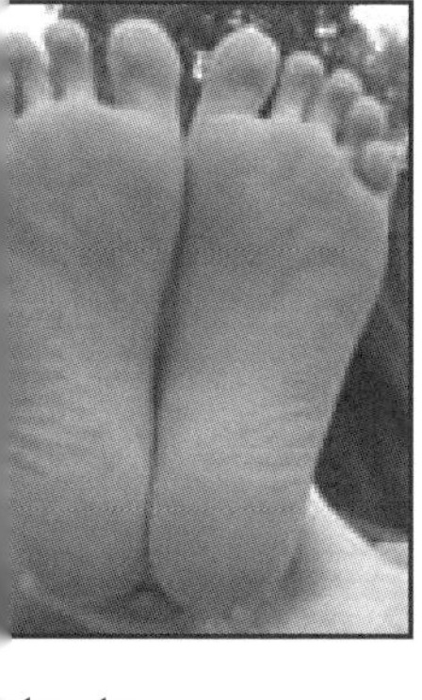

tnote

It takes a bit of practice to get the "feel" of a good gynaecoid pelvis.

APPENDIX 5

MATERNITY REFLEXOLOGY CLIENT QUESTIONNAIRE

Name: Date of Birth:

Address: Tel:

EDD: No. Weeks pregnant on first visit:

Do you have an obstetric caregiver? Obstetrician / GP / Midwife

Name: Contact No. / Address

Does your obstetrician / GP / midwife know that you are receiving reflexology? Yes / No

1. THIS PREGNANCY:

Is this a planned pregnancy? Yes / No

Was this pregnancy conceived naturally? Yes / No

Is this your first pregnancy? Yes / No
(If not please complete section 2.)

Have you had a scan? Yes / No

If 'yes', was it allright? Yes / No

In addition to routine tests, have you had or will you have other tests? Amniocentesis
Glucose Tolerance Test
Other

Do you have or are you suffering from the following?

Backache	Yes / No	R
Rib pain	Yes / No	R
Symphysis pubis pain	Yes / No	R
Groin pain	Yes / No	O
Braxton Hicks contractions	Yes / No	O
Vaginal bleeding	Yes / No	O
Morning sickness	Yes / No	Y
Heartburn	Yes / No	Y
Food fads	Yes / No	Y
Constipation	Yes / No	Y
Diarrhoea	Yes / No	Y
Frequency of Micturition	Yes / No	L
Cystitis	Yes / No	L
Protein, sugar or blood in the urine	Yes / No	L
Palpitations	Yes / No	G
Anaemia	Yes / No	G
Leg pain/cramp	Yes / No	G

Varicose veins	Yes / No	G
Deep Vein Thrombosis	Yes / No	G
Haemorrhoids	Yes / No	G
Low blood pressure	Yes / No	G
High blood pressure	Yes / No	G
Oedema	Yes / No	T
Panic attacks	Yes / No	B
Carpal tunnel syndrome	Yes / No	I
Sciatica	Yes / No	I
Headaches	Yes / No	I
Stretch marks	Yes / No	V
Itchy skin	Yes / No	V
Tender breasts	Yes / No	V
Fatigue	Yes / No	P
Diabetes	Yes / No	P
Mood swings	Yes / No	M
Insomnia	Yes / No	M

Initials indicate colour in the Maternity Reflexology Pregnancy Care Reference cards.
Red, Orange, Yellow, Lime, Green, Turquoise, Blue, Indigo, Violet, Purple, Magenta

2. PREVIOUS PREGNANCIES:

Have you suffered any miscarriages? Yes / No

Have you had any terminations of pregnancy? Yes / No

How many previous pregnancies?	1	2	3	4
Was the pregnancy normal?				
Did you suffer any of the above ailments?				
Was the baby: Pre-term.... on time…. overdue?				
Was the delivery normal?				
Were you induced?				
Did you have an epidural?				
Was the delivery assisted i.e. forceps, suction?				
Did you have stitches?				
Did you breast feed?				
Did you have any postnatal problems?				

OTHER NOTES:

APPENDIX 6

LIST OF MATERNITY REFLEXOLOGY RELATED PUBLISHED RESEARCH PAPERS & ARTICLES

AoR Guidelines for Pregnant Clients, 2002 September, Reflexions

Bird, Adam, et al, 1997, *A Prospective Investigation of the Effects of Pregnancy on Footprint Parameters*

Brown, Sarah, 2001 September, *Reflexology in Pregnancy and Childbirth,* Reflexions

Car, Rachel 2001 December, *My Birth Story - Reflexology Style*, Reflexions

Clausen, Jette Aaroe and Møller Else, 1996, *Foot Reflex Therapy in the Treatment of Primary Inertia During Labour,* International Confederation of Midwives 24th Triennial Congress, Oslo

Copley Ester, 1999 March, *Reflexology and Infertility: Two Case Studies,* Foot Prints

Croser, Helen, 2000 September, *Reflexology in the Special Care Nursery - Pt 2*, Footprints

Cutler, Sarah-Ellen 2002 September, *A Stress Free Pregnancy,* Reflexions

Evans Margarita 1990 Jan, *Reflex Zone Therapy for Mothers,* Nursing Times

Enzer, Susanne, 2001, *Endocrine Balance,* Reflexology World

Feter, E., Bering, L., Lenstrup, C., Roseno, H., & Taxbol, D., 1988, *Reflexology in Relation to Birth*. Proceedings of the 23rd International Confederation of Midwives Congress, Vancouver, Canada. Vol. 2

Fransen, Peter Lund, 2000, *Why Does Reflexology Work? Is the Explanation Found in the Embryo?,* 4th European Conference RIEN

Green, Elizabeth 1996 Sept, *Treating Hypertension and Pre-Eclampsia at Queen Charlottes,* Reflections

Holt, Jane, 2000 March, *Case Study: Reflexology and Fertility,* Reflexions

Krogsgaard, Dorthe, 1999 March, *Treating Colic in Infants,* Foot Prints

Kruchik-Biderman, Moshe 2001 December, *The Use of Reflexology in Childbirth,* Reflexology World

Leiser, Bernadette, 2000 June, *Carpel Tunnel Syndrome in Pregnancy,* Reflexology World

Liisberg, Gabriella Bering, 1983, *Reflexology and Childbirth,* Forenede Danske Zoneterapeuter

Motha, Gowrie and McGrath, Jane 1994, *The Effects of Reflexology on Labour Outcome,* Association of Reflexologists. Reflexology Research Reports (2nd ed). Association of Reflexologists, London

Motha, Gowrie and Papakonstantinou, Katrina, 1997 Sept, *Pregnancy,* Reflexions

Nagasu, Chikako, 2001 June, *Reflexology in the Fields of Obstetrics and Gynaecology,* Reflexology World

Olivari Danila, 1998, *Passo dopo passo nella gestazione,* Reflessologia Oggi

Oleson, Terry, & Flocco, William, 1993 Dec, *Randomized Controlled Study of Premenstrual Symptoms Treated with Ear, Hand and Foot Reflexology,* Obstetrics & Gynaecology Vol.82, No 6

Pankhurst, Daisy2002 September, *Case Profile - Pregnancy & Childbirth,* Reflexions

Rawji, Zia 1994 Dec, *Aspirations: a Picture of the Project,* Reflexions

Siu-Lan Li and Cai-Xia Shu, 1996, *Galactagogue Effect of Foot Reflexology in 217 Parturient Women,* 1996 Beijing International Reflexology Conference

Sorrig, Kirsten, 1988 July, *Easier Births Using Reflexology,* Berlingske Tidende

Spilby, Helen, 1993 Feb, *Giving Complementary Therapy with Midwifery Care for the 1990s,* Midwives Chronical & Nursing Notes

Surukka, Tiina, 1998 Sept, *How to Measure the Effectiveness of Reflexology as a Labour Pain Killer?* Third European Conference of Reflexology Tampere, Finland

Thompson, Nicole, 2001, *My Reflexology Diary,* Reflexology World

Tiran, Denise, 1996, *The Use of Complementary Therapies in Midwifery Practice: A Focus on Reflexology,* Complementary Therapies in Nursing and Midwifery. 2

Warren, Helen, 1997 June, *Working with Premature Babies,* Reflexology World

Wilson, Anne, 1995 March, *A Case of Feet,* ACMI Journal

APPENDIX 7

SOME OBSERVATIONS ABOUT SUB-FERTILITY FROM REFLEXOLOGISTS

1. SUB-FERTILITY / REFLEXOLOGY AND THYROID FUNCTION

Contributed by Anne Thomas, Cornwall UK

Imbalances in the thyroid reflex zones

"In many of the cases of sub-fertility with which I have worked I have often discovered imbalances in the thyroid reflexes - leading in particular to a suspicion of low thyroid function. Some common symptoms of low thyroid function include no ovulation, a short luteal phase (which means that any fertilized egg is not sustained in its early phase for long enough) and sometimes an increase in the hormone prolactin - an excess of which has a negative impact on pregnancy. Additionally, the adrenal glands will often seem low in energy; adrenal insufficiency can go hand-in-hand with low thyroid function, which can further complicate diagnosis and treatment.

Working the thyroid reflex

On working the thyroid reflex directly this would often feel hard and dry and there would often be lumps/calluses in the area between zones 1 and 2 metatarsals and around the base of the ball of the foot in zone 1 - for some practitioners this area is indicated as a secondary/helper thyroid reflex. My experience is leading me to suspect that the more this latter area is calloused, the more chronic the condition is. Even a quick visual check on these areas can set alarm bells ringing. Checking with the client would often produce a list of symptoms consistent with hypothyroidism: low energy/tired all the time; feeling constantly cold; dry skin/hair - sometimes with the hair falling out; inability to lose weight; depression/feeling tearful.

One client

In one particular client with a young son of 2 years old and a seeming inability to fall pregnant again, the thyroid reflex was very hard and dry with calluses presenting as above. Additionally she had all the above symptoms so I suggested she requested blood tests for thyroid function. Her GP was quite supportive and in her case, the tests came back demonstrating hypothyroidism and she was immediately put on thyroxin - the standard medication, which is a synthetic version of the hormone naturally produced by the thyroid gland. In the meanwhile she continued having reflexology. Two weeks after she started her medication she delightedly reported that she was pregnant but sadly miscarried at 8 weeks. This led me to consider several possibilities:

Possibilities

1. That reflexology had already begun to allow the thyroid gland to rebalance to some degree

2. That reflexology had 'primed' the body to some extent so that when the synthetic thyroxin was administered it was used efficiently right from the start

3. That possible adrenal insufficiency had not been investigated

My belief

Obviously there are always other possibilities. However, I believe the miscarriage occurred because she fell pregnant too early and her body (in particular thyroid and/or adrenal glands) was still not sufficiently balanced to carry the pregnancy to term.

A second client

A second client volunteered as a guinea pig for one of my students on my professional reflexology course. She had fallen pregnant following participation in a trial investigating the benefits of reflexology in infertility and was 12 weeks pregnant at the time of her first treatment in class.
After an in-depth discussion with the volunteer student and me, the client proceeded with her treatment.
Through visual assessment the student immediately recognised a potential imbalance in the thyroid reflexes and palpation of both the thyroid and adrenal gland reflexes suggested low energy.

Experience

This latter experience in particular has suggested to me that to discontinue treatment during the first trimester of pregnancy is not in the client's best interest, particularly where there has potentially been low thyroid/adrenal function.
The reflexology might have raised the levels sufficiently to allow conception, but if the reflexology is stopped it is possible that function might drop back again and create a risk to the developing foetus.
I personally believe it is vital to continue with reflexology throughout the pregnancy so long as the client has been receiving reflexology prior to or at least during the preconception phase."

2. COFFEE / COLA LEGS

Contributed by Val Groome, Essex, UK

Coffee / cola legs	*"When I start a reflexology treatment I hold the heels in the palms of my hands so that my fingers go slightly up the back of the legs. When I can see swelling and feel a sponginess, I call it 'coffee / cola legs'. This condition is often present when sub-fertility is a problem.*
The area	*The area where this is normally found is above the point where the back of the shoe (shoe line) touches the leg. Instead of a shapely leg going up to the calf, the leg is swollen and feels spongy. The tissue below the shoe line will not be spongy, swollen or puffy.*
Caution	*If there is oedema around the foot and ankle the cause may be more serious.*
Questions	*Why does this strange effect happen? Why does this irregularity stop at the shoe line? Why doesn't this show on the dorsal aspect of the foot? I haven't got a clue! I have asked many medical people and they do not know.*
My observations	*Through feeling, observing and questioning my clients I have reached my conclusion that the common denominators are coffee, cola, Earl grey tea, or Assam tea. I also suspect some herbal and green teas also cause this effect.*
Solution	*By cutting out the offending fluids slowly (to avoid withdrawal symptoms) and by having regular reflexology treatments the legs do change shape. If clients continue to drink coffee etc. even though they are having reflexology treatments the legs do not change shape.*
I believe	*I believe "coffee / cola" legs can be a problem in all ages, from small children to the very elderly. The condition aggravates many other health problems such as: pre-eclampsia, arthritis, rheumatoid arthritis, mood swings, Chron's disease, colitis, headaches, obesity, and lethargy to name but a few. I have found that in the majority of cases, replacing these fluids with water, detoxification takes place - encouraging health to improve.*
Success	*I am extremely pleased with my success in sub-fertility and I will continue researching toxins that could be detrimental to fertility and other health problems."*

APPENDIX 8

MY PREGNANT FEET - MELISSA'S STORY

Contributed by Melissa Cooney
Melissa Cooney was a reflexology student in my course Advanced Reflexology in 1997.

The following is her project presentation. It is so beautiful and poignant that I print it here unedited and offer heartfelt thanks to Melissa.

"What I put forward to you this afternoon is not what I have been trained to do. I have a background in Science and that training reflects in almost everything I do in my life: objective opinions based on research. My most recent "adventure" is put to you from a subjective point of view, with the Left Brain attempting to rationalise and turn my experience into a logical acceptance.

November 22, 1996

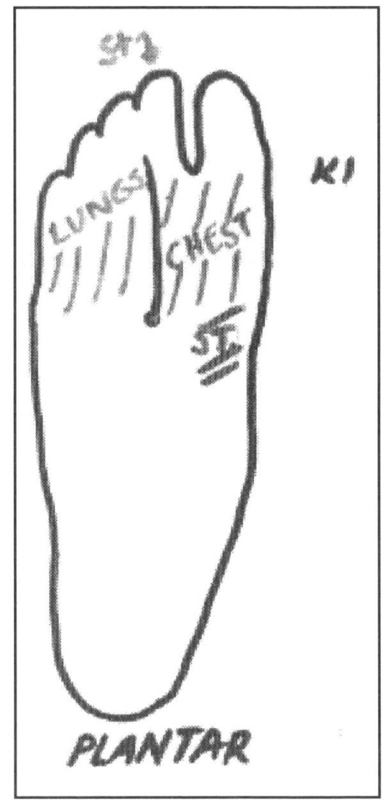

We had been looking forward to adding a "critter" as hubby so affectionately calls it, to our lives for quite a while now. Finding out that we were pregnant was a joyful moment in our lives, and being the conscientious reflexology student that I am, I started taking notice of changes in my body and in our mind set that might reflect in our feet.

Looking back I suppose I should have realised that there was definitely something different about my body. In the past two weeks or so there have been signs in my feet that I feel respond to early pregnancy. In fact, there has been an increase in my internal conversation, with Left Brain (LB) rationalising the thoughts and intuitions that Right Brain (RB) has had. Then there were the itches in my feet that travelled from Kidney 1 (K1) point directly up the border of longitudinal zone 2 and 3.

LB said that it was just the fact that I had bought 4 new pairs of shoes and wasn't used to wearing them. RB was saying that there was a change in my energy levels. Not having done all the Chinese based reflexology, LB now recognises it as gathering of Pre-natal Ch'i. The path of energy flow corresponded so closely to the concept that Pre-natal Ch'i, or all heredity of Life Energy, begins in the kidneys and moves to the Gate of Life (navel), then upward to the digestive system, where Kidney Ch'i joins with Grain Ch'i, and then upwards to join with Air Ch'i.

The energy level changes within my body reflected very closely. My feet were itchy at K1 point, and the line of energy went through the diaphragm line, throughout the reflection of lungs and then up to the second toe, and over to the longitudinal zone 2 and 3 border, where stomach meridian lies.

Personally I thought I had some sort of stomach virus. I found that I couldn't handle milk and coffee, the smell of lamb or greasy foods any more. My stomach felt as though it was actually fluttering, and I had felt the need for fruits and raw vegetables, so much so that I actually consumed a mango, a kiwi fruit, a punnet of strawberries, a peach and a litre and a half of filtered water in the space of an hour (and in front of my senior class, who looked at me as if I was possessed!). LB now says that it was the rising Kidney Ch'i joining with Grain Ch'i, and the altering levels of energy corresponded commencing from about six hours after conception. I now know that the second toe also represents thoughts regarding feelings, I, we were definitely awaiting the arrival of a new soul into our lives with anticipation and excitement. The changes in my feet in the past few weeks made logical sense. Thank you LB.

November 29, 1996

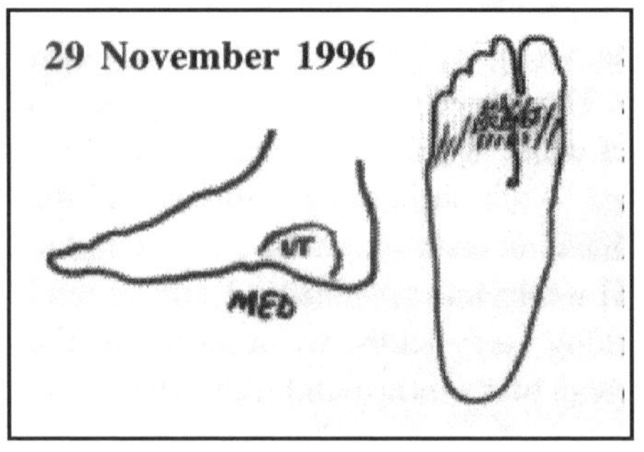

Subject to scrutiny from the reflexology class, my feet presented with an early maternal pattern, that is, changes to the uterus reflection, and a continued increase in energy levels - but that is not all. My breast area on my feet had become a little more red, swollen and sensitive. As was its anatomical reflection! The energy path along the Kidney meridian was still going strong, but I was becoming tired. My feet reflected this every time I sat or lay down - they definitely flopped over, too tired to hold themselves up!

December 8, 1996

A small amount of bleeding occurred, and a little panic.

December 9, 1996

More bleeding, more panic, and off to hospital. Spent the day in hospital on a drip. Underwent ultrasounds - no body was visible, but size of gestational sac indicates 5.5 weeks. No major problem detected, discharged. Blood tests and urine analysis also conducted - no abnormalities were found.

December 10, 1996

Continued bleeding, blood tests and sent to bed until December 19 1996. "Just a safety precaution" I was told, "you've had a threatened miscarriage". That was it, the news I didn't want to hear. Did as I was told, and went to bed. Blood tests taken - and normal HCG levels found.

December 11, 1996

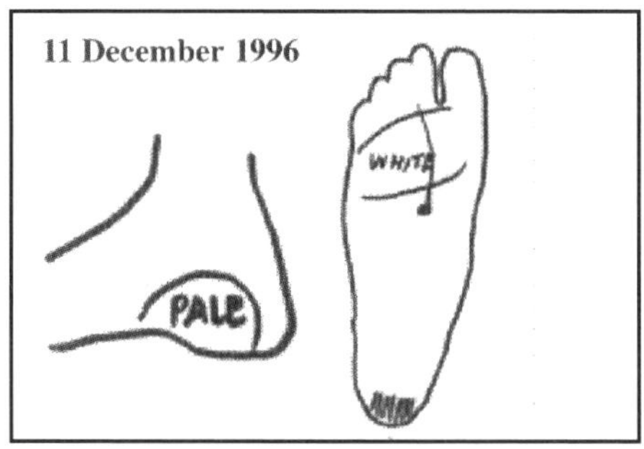

Husband drove me to class, picked up literature and went home. Feeling pretty useless actually. Not used to being told to stop and do nothing. I was frightened not to. We wanted this soul and fear had set in. Typical RB stuff.

My heels had coloured red, my chest area was white and my uterus area was pale, almost white. My stability and sense of security (my heel) was threatened, my mobility was stifled, I was frightened and fed up, and my reproductive organs were obviously tired. Makes sense, considering. Thanks LB.

December 18, 1996

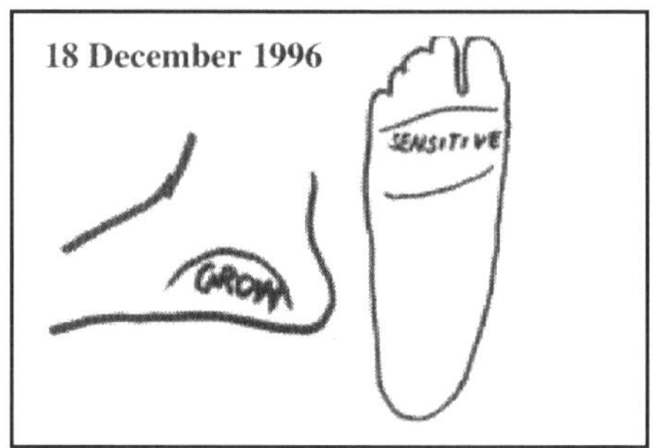

A lot of time spent sleeping and soul searching. However, I was feeling much better, my chest area was flaking (irritable at heart for not being able to do anything to help my situation and sick of feeling like an invalid).

My feet still show signs of pregnancy. The uterus area was obviously swelling, reflecting the growth of my womb. My chest area also felt tingly, and the pressure of shoes on them felt like my feet (and breasts) were being constricted.

December 19, 1996 to January 13, 1997

My feet continued to swell in the appropriate places, but my uterus area remains pale and white. LB said that of course it would, being pregnant for the first time was an unusual state for my body, and all nutrients were sent there first as a priority. The path of energy up the Kidney meridian had stopped, and to be honest, apart from tender breasts, I felt no different than I had previously.

January 13, 1997

The appointment with the obstetrician, our first, was an exciting and heart-wrenching day all in one. The obstetrician was running late, so we went for lunch and then a walk, window-shopping. Bought a beautiful cane basinet. Returned to the obstetrician's office, and the news was not good. After examination and discussion, I was found to be a little on the small side for 11 weeks into pregnancy. An ultrasound was decided upon. To cut a long story short, we returned to the obstetrician an hour or so later with blank ultrasound films. Placenta - fine, Amniotic sac - fine...baby none. A few tears, but preparations for hospitalisation had to be made. Didn't want to go home. We stayed out until midnight and didn't go to bed until 3.30 am. didn't sleep at all.

January 14, 1997

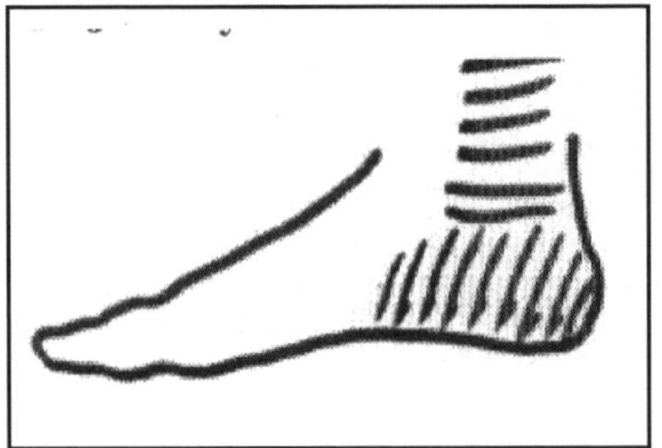

An early morning procedure with a team of specialists that I had never seen in my life. No time for trepidation, things have to be done and over with. LB.

After the procedure and back in the ward, I looked down at my feet. True! Sounds strange but I was interested to see how our loss affected my feet. The whole pelvic area was red, from my bladder area to the back of the heel, and even around my ankles, where it also felt like I had been given a Chinese burn.

January 16, 1997

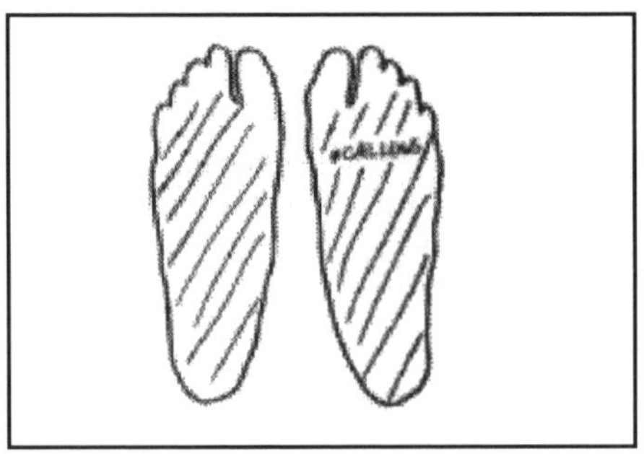

Felt like a robot. Found myself walking through Woolworth's with no smile. Now that worried me. Postnatal depression, if I can claim that, set in. RB won over and my emotions let loose. The whole of the soles of my feet were red, and over my heart area a small callous had developed. My feet remained this way for at least a week, and then they started to peel, not just in small sections, but in sheets. To me this reflected the process of realising the idea that we had had about being pregnant.

January 21, 1997

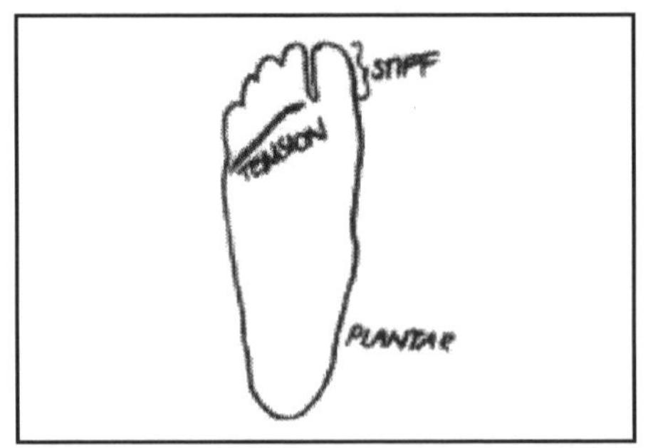

The most severe migraine that I had ever experienced set in, and lasted for 10 days. You guessed it my feet reflected this also. My big toe felt as though I had tried to kick a brick, and my trapezes area was rigid, as was the flexibility of my metatarsals. Eventually, after trying migraine medication and then massage, it went. The sadness in our hearts is still there, but acceptance has set in.

February 7, 1997

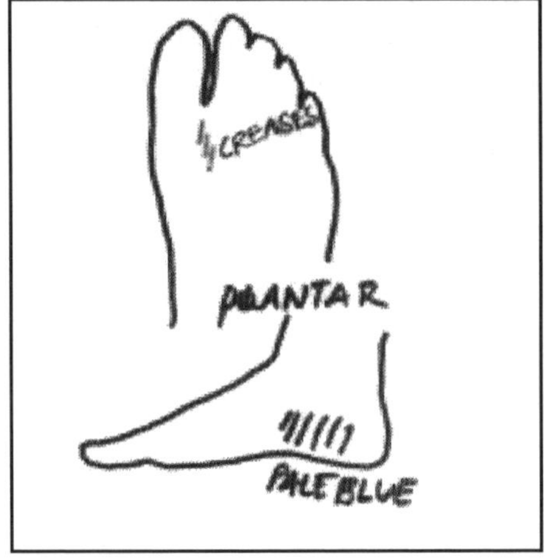

Yes I gave my feet a close inspection last night. I found that my reproductive area is a pale blue, and my heart area has a crease through it that I had not noticed before. Bruised emotions, and a small tear in my heart, a feeling of sadness and a few tears in my eyes are present at the moment. With time, I am sure both will fade, but not quite."

Bibliography

Allan V. J., 1994, *Oceans of Streams,* Om Shiatsu Centre

Bauer C., 1987, *Acupressure for Women,* The Crossing Press

Berkson D., 1977, *The Foot Book,* Harper Perennial.

Bird A. R. et al, 1999, *A Prospective Investigation of the Effects of Pregnancy on the Footprint Parameters,* Journal of the American Podiatric Medical Association.

Blake C. F. 1994 spring, Vol. 19, *Foot-binding in Neo-Confucian China and the Appropriation of Female Labour Signs.*

Enzer S. 2000, *Reflexology a Tool for Midwives,* Soul to Sole Reflexology.

Goody J. 1990, *The Oriental, the Ancient and the Primitive,* Cambridge University Press.

Johari H. 1996, *Ayurvedic Massage,* Healing Arts Press.

Judith A. 1994, *Wheels of Life,* Llewellyn's New Worlds.

Kapit W. & Elson L., 1997, *The Anatomy Colouring Book,* Harper & Rowe, Publishers

Kirkup J. *The Foot You Never Knew.*

Levy H. S. 1992, *The Lotus Lovers: The Complete History of the Curious Erotic Custom of Foot-binding in China,* Prometheus Books.

Mackie G. 1996 Dec Vol. 61, *Ending Foot-binding and Infibulation; a Convention Account,* American Sociological Review.

Mackereth P. A. & Tiran D., 2002, *Clinical Reflexology, a Guide for Health Professionals,* Churchill Livingstone.

Meridian Therapy Course Notes, 1997.

Naish F. & Roberts J., 1997, *The Natural Way to Better Babies, Preconception Health Care for Prospective Parents,* Random House.

Naish F. & Roberts J., 1999, *The Natural Way to a Better Pregnancy,* Doubleday.

NSW Health Department, 1994, *Pregnancy Care,* State Health Publication No. (HPA) 970085.

Page C., 1992, *Frontiers of Health, from Healing to Wholeness,* C. W. Daniel Company Ltd.

Reid E., and Enzer S., 1997, *Maternity Reflexology a Guide for Reflexologists,* Born to be Free & Soul to Sole Reflexology.

Rossi W. 1976, *The Sex Life of the Foot and Shoe,* Kreiger Publishing Company.

Saint-Pierre G. & Shapiro D. 2000, *The Metamorphic Technique,* Viga.

Sharamon S. & Baginski B. 1991, *The Chakra Handbook,* Lotus Light Publication.

Stanjyo Y., 1985, *Chinese Massage Course Notes.*

Sweet B. with Tiran D., 1997, *Mayes' Midwifery a Textbook for Midwives,* Baillière Tindall, 12th edition

Tai D., 1987, *Acupuncture and Moxibustion,* Harper Rowe.

Tiwari M. 1995, *Ayurveda Secrets of Healing,* Lotus Press.

Translated by Tay G., and Eu Hoi Khaw, 1988, *The Rwo Shur Health Method,* Gerdine Co.

Yelland S., 1996, *Acupuncture in Midwifery,* Books for Midwives Press

Recommended Reading

A Case of Feet, 1995 March, Anne Wilson, ACMI Journal

Hands of Light, a Guide to Healing Through the Human Energy Field, 1988, Barbara Ann Brennan.

Pregnancy Care, by The NSW Health Department

Reflexology and Premature Babies, 2000, Helen Croser. Chapter 7 Reflexology a Tool for Midwives.

Reflexology in the Special Care Nursery - Part 2, 2000 Sept, Helen Croser, Reflexology Association of Australia magazine FootPrints.

Reflexology a Tool for Midwives, 2000, Susanne Enzer

The Lunar Cycle, a Guide to Natural Fertility Control, 1989, Francesca Naish

The Metamorphic Technique, Principles and Practice, 2000, Gaston Saint-Pierre and Debby Shapiro

The Metamorphic Technique with Gaston Saint-Pierre. AoR members' seminars *"Types of Birth and the Way if Affects Us"*. The transcript is in Reflexions March 2003 Issue 70.

The Natural Way to Better Babies, Preconception Health Care for Prospective Parents, reprint 1997, Francesca Naish & Jeanette Roberts

*The Natural Way to Better Pregnancy,*1999, Francesca Naish & Jeanette Roberts

The Sex Life of the Foot and Shoe, 1976, William Rossi

The Wild Genie, 2001, Alexandra Pope

Treating Colic in Infants, 1999 March, Dorthe Krogsgaard, Reflexology Association of Australia magazine FootPrints.

Vertical Reflexology, Lynne Booth

Wheels of Life - a Users Guide to the Chakra System, 1994, Anodea Judith

Working with Premature Babies, 199,7 June Helen Warren, Edited version of a presentation at the 1996 RAA Conference in Sydney, Reflexology World

Resources

Video	*The Hormone Hat, the Effects of the Female Hormones of Fertility,* by Susanne Enzer, Grannie-Su Enterprises.
Reference cards	*Maternity Reflexology Pregnancy Care Reference cards,* by Soul to Sole Reflexology.

Indexes

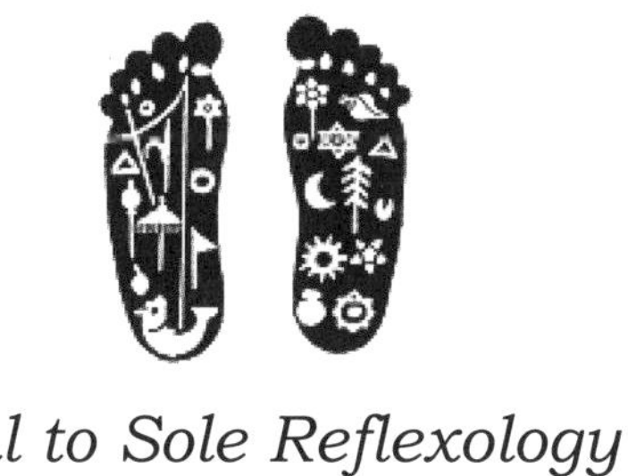

Soul to Sole Reflexology

Index of Pregnancy Conditions, Minor Ailments & Major Problems

Index of Postnatal Conditions

Index of Baby Conditions

Index of Menstrual Cycle Problems

Index of Reflexology Techniques